Cholesterol Cookbook for a Healthy Heart

25 Heart Friendly Recipes

Your Gift

I wanted to show my appreciation that you support my work so I've put together a free gift for you.

http://bonusfreebook.org/

Just visit the link above to download it now.

I know you will love this gift.

If you like this book, you can see and buy my other books on this link:

All books **Jessica Huston here**

Thank you for attention!

With love,

Jessica Huston

Table of Contents

Introduction

Cholesterol is the word that has been associated with lots of negativity. It has gained notorious fame due to its linkage to multiple heart diseases. However, it is LDL (Low-density lipoprotein) cholesterol known as "bad cholesterol" that we really need to be worried about when it comes to our diet.

To lower cholesterol levels we must follow a few simple guidelines. There are some foods that need to be consumed sufficiently, while some foods should be consumed as much as possible. Pork, beef, lamb and whole-milk dairy products need to be consumed moderately given their high fat content. Other foods containing high saturated fats such as margarine, butter, lard, palm, kernel, and coconut oil are also on this list. Sausages, bacon, burgers, and kebabs, pastries, cakes, pies, rich creamy desserts, and biscuits also in a restricted list and need to be consumed as less as possible.

A low cholesterol diet includes many ingredients with a healthy amount of omega-3, omega-6, and omega-9 fatty acids. They control our cholesterol levels and greatly help you in leading a healthy lifestyle. Foods derived from plants have negligible or no cholesterol at all. Heart friendly ingredients with low cholesterol like legumes, seeds, vegetables, fruits, nuts, and whole, unprocessed grains should be included more in the diet for healthy heart functions.

Vegetables, fruit and nuts (avocados, coconuts, olives, seeds, etc.) have also good, healthy fats making them ideal to include in our diet. Another reason to include fruits and vegetables in your low cholesterol diet is that they contain the high amount of antioxidants. Antioxidants help a lot in preventing the circulating cholesterol from oxidizing. When cholesterol oxidizes, it damages our heart health. Fruits and vegetables also supply our body with phytosterols and bind with bad cholesterol within the intestines. Thus, they minimize its absorption.

Seeds (sunflower, sesame, pumpkin, and flax seeds), oils (sesame, flax, pumpkin, sunflower, and olive), avocados, and nuts (walnuts, almonds, pistachios, and macadamias) are very rich in phytosterols to keep our health healthy. All vegetables, legumes, and fruit, that are rich in fiber, help in the excretion of cholesterol by attaching to unwanted fat in our body. Healthy ingredients that are rich in soluble and insoluble fiber are chickpeas, beans, lentils, oatmeal, flaxseed, citrus fruits, barley, brown rice, strawberries, and Brussels sprouts.

Modest portions of lean meat and poultry are healthy for our heart; also soya foods, white and oily fish, and low fat dairy products are rich with essential nutrients and saturated fats also play an important role in maintaining a healthy cholesterol level.

This book is a special collection of 25 Low Cholesterol recipes divided into the versatile categories of main course meals, seafood recipes, soups, desserts, and drinks. Each recipe has been smartly formed by including a smart combination of ingredients to minimize the level of bad cholesterol and increase the level of good cholesterol in your body. The recipes are high in fiber and vitamins; they are greatly helpful to keep your cholesterol numbers in the safe zone.

Get ready to make some healthy changes in your routine diet. Let's get started!

Chapter 1: Super Healthy Seafood Recipes

1) Salmon Zucchini Kebabs

Prep Time: 25-30 mins

Serves: 4

Ingredients:

- 1 cup cherry tomatoes
- 6 skinless salmon fillets, cut into 1 inch pieces
- 2 shallots, ends trimmed, halved
- 2 zucchinis, make small cubes
- 3 limes, make thin wedges

Directions:

- Preheat barbecue or char grill over medium-high heat.

- Thread the fish cubes onto skewers; now gently thread zucchinis, shallots, and tomatoes.

- Repeat to make 10-12 skewers.

- Grill for about 3-4 minutes each side.

- Transfer to a plate, cover with foil and set aside for 5 minutes.

- Take off the foil and serve warm!

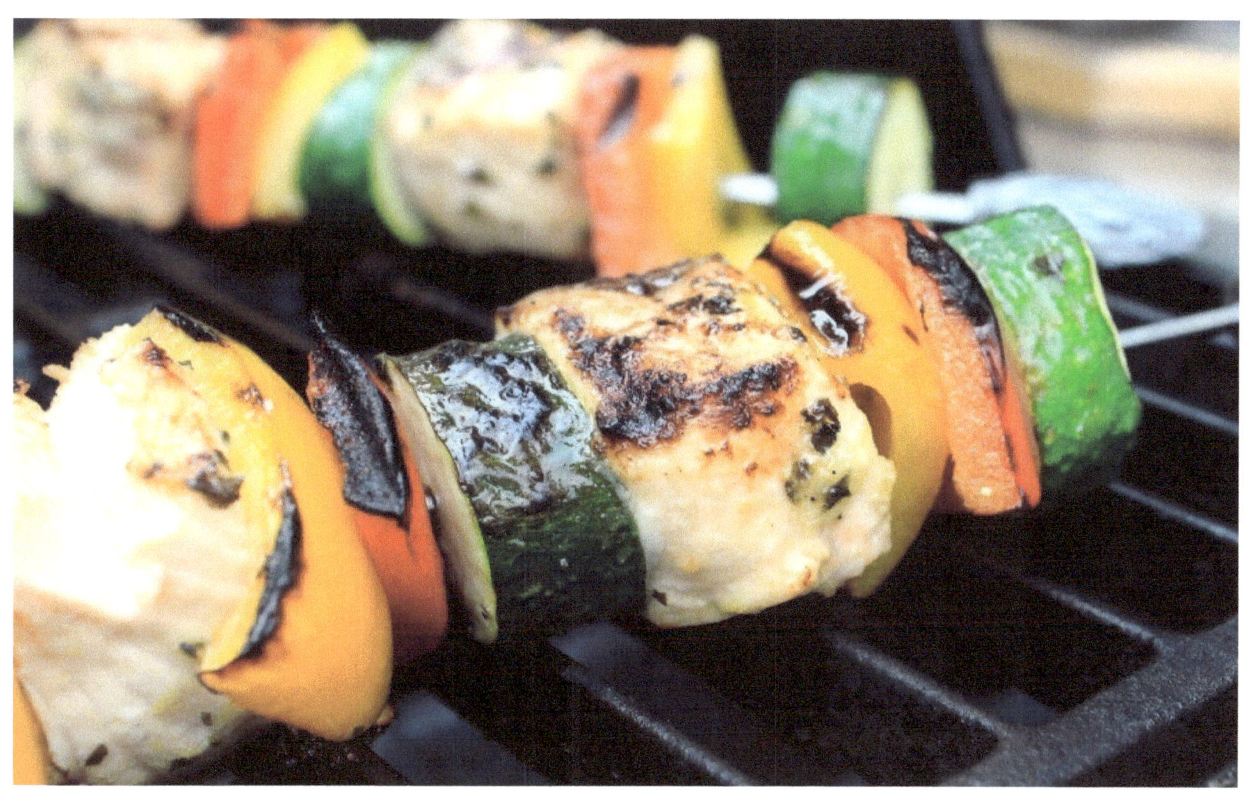

2)Quinoa Bean Salmon Bowl

Prep Time: 20-25 mins

Serves:4

Ingredients:

- 2 cups cooked and flaked salmon
- 1/2 red bell pepper, chopped
- 1/2 cup canned beans, drained
- 1/2 cup quinoa, rinsed
- 1 cups water
- 1 tbs. extra virgin olive oil
- 6 green onions, chopped
- 1 tsp. Dijon mustard
- 1 tsp. lemon juice
- 3 tbs.parsley leaves, finely cut
- black pepper, to taste

Directions:

- Boil quinoa in one cup of water for 15 minutes in a pan.

- Fluff with a fork and set aside.

- In a large mixing bowl mix: salmon, bell pepper, onions, parsley, mustard, olive oil and lemon juice.

- Mix in the quinoa. Season with pepper and toss to combine.

- Serve and enjoy!

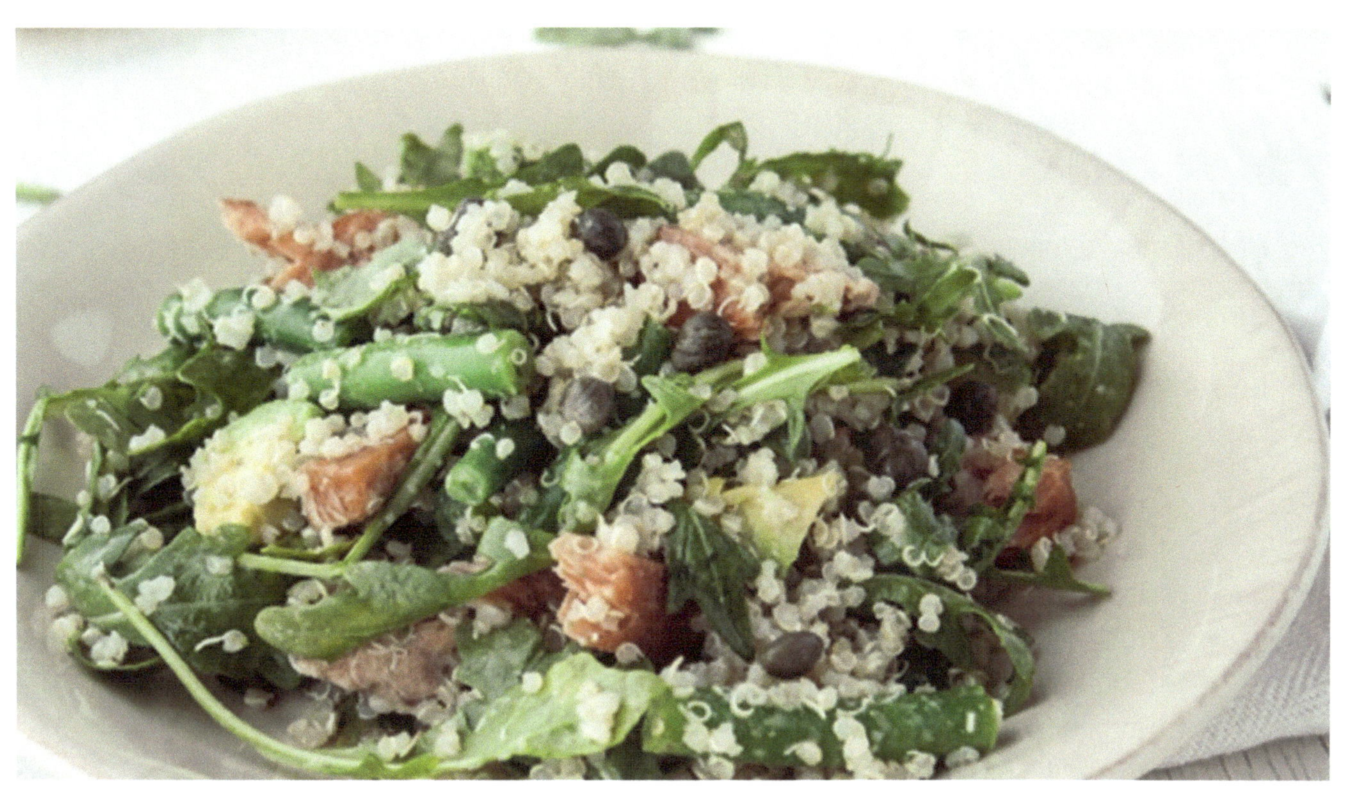

3)Salmon Asparagus Salad

Prep Time: 5 mins

Serves:3-4

Ingredients:

- 1 bunch asparagus, trimmed, cut into 2 inch pieces
- 1 can salmon, drained and make large chunks
- 1 cup corn kernels, cooked
- 4 tbs. lemon juice
- 2 tbs. olive oil, extra virgin
- 1 cucumber, peeled and chopped
- 1 avocado, peeled and cubed
- 1 tbs. dill, very finely chopped

Directions:

- Cook a sparagus in boiling salted water for 2-3 minutes.

- Drain the water and pat dry.

- Mix the asparagus, cucumber, avocado, corn, and salmon into a mixing bowl.

- In a small bowl, whisk some lemon juice, olive oil, and dill.

- Mix in salt and black pepper to taste.

- Pour over the salad, toss well and serve!

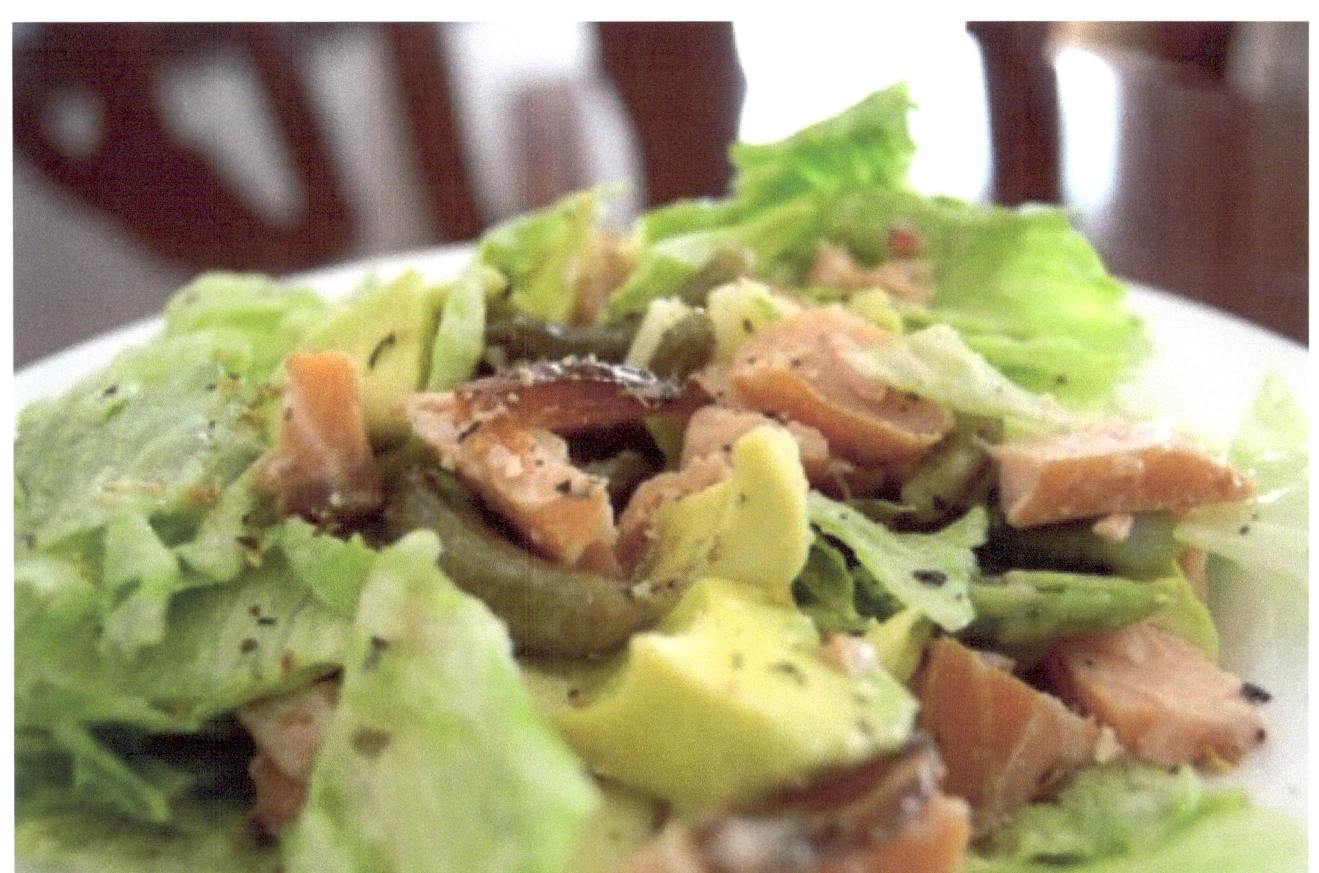

4) White Wine Sea Bass

Prep Time: 25-30 mins

Serves: 3-4

Ingredients:

- 1 pound scaled sea bass
- 10 black olives, pitted and halved
- 3 lemon wedges
- 5 oz. fennel, trimmed and sliced
- 6 spring onions, chopped
- 2 garlic cloves, chopped
- ½ tsp. paprika
- ½ cup dry white wine
- 3 tbs. extra virgin olive oil
- 1 tbs. capers
- 2 garlic cloves, finely chopped
- Pepper and salt to taste

Directions:

- Take a mixing bowl, mix in: pepper, olive oil, garlic, and salt.

- Arrange fennel in a shallow ovenproof casserole.

- Add onions and add fish on top.

- Pour over the olive mixture.

- Spread olives, paprika, and lemon wedges over and top with some wine over.

- Cover the dish with a foil and bake for 20 minutes.

- Serve warm!

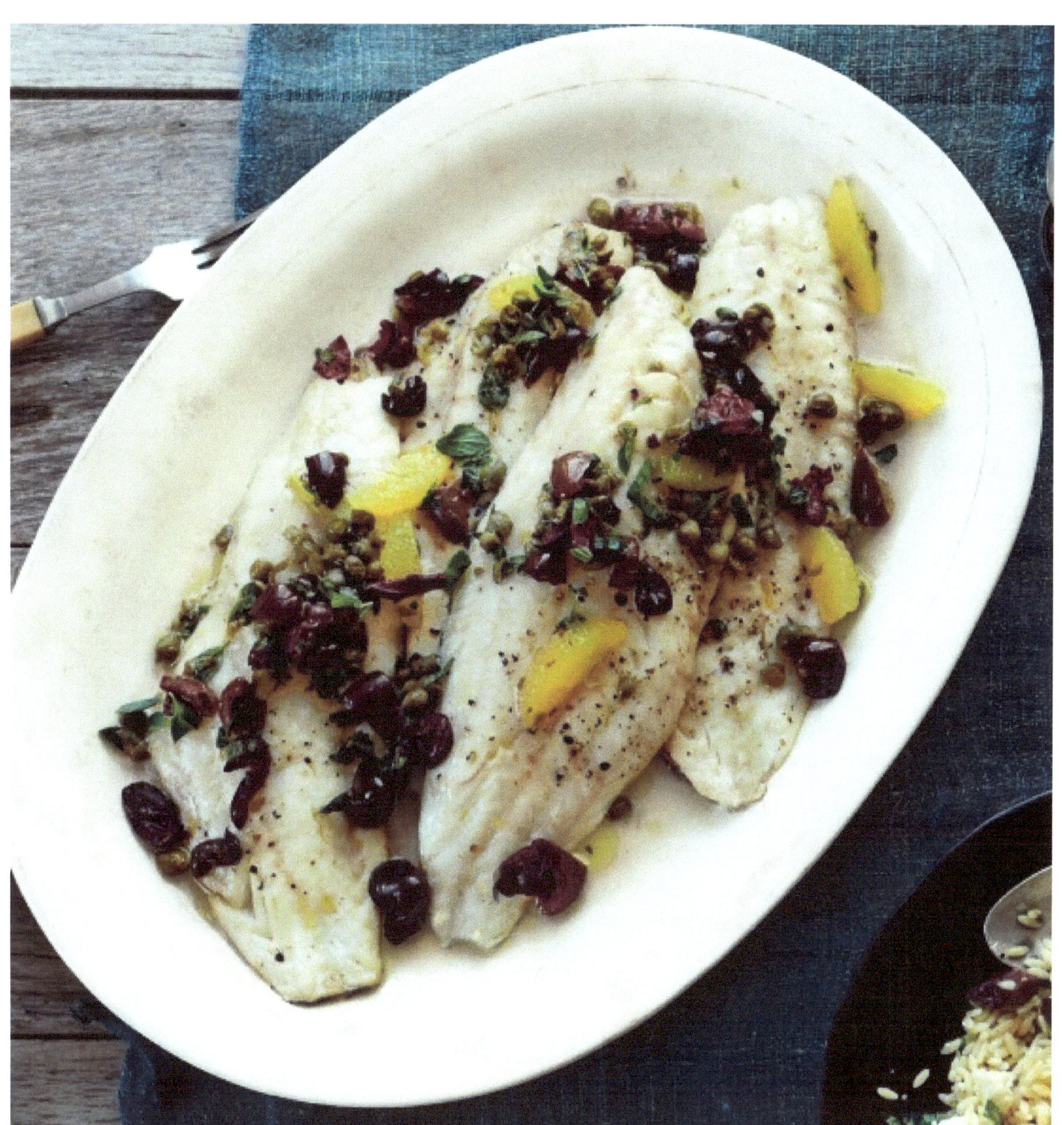

5) Spinach Baked Fillets

Prep Time: 10 mins

Serves: 4

Ingredients:

- 4 tbs. breadcrumbs
- 2 tbs. lemon zest
- 4 white fish fillets
- 1 tbs. rosemary, dried
- 1 tsp. garlic powder
- 2 tbs. extra virgin olive oil
- 1 tsp. salt

Directions:

- Mix rosemary, breadcrumbs, lemon zest, garlic powder and salt in a food processor and blend until all the ingredients are well combined.

- Arrange the fillets, skin-side up, on a lined baking tray.

- Grill them for 3-4 minutes.

- Turn the fish over and gently press 1/4 of the breadcrumb mixture over the top of each fillet.

- Top with some olive oil and grill for 4 minutes until the crust is golden and the fish is flaked well.

- Serve warm with steamed spinach.

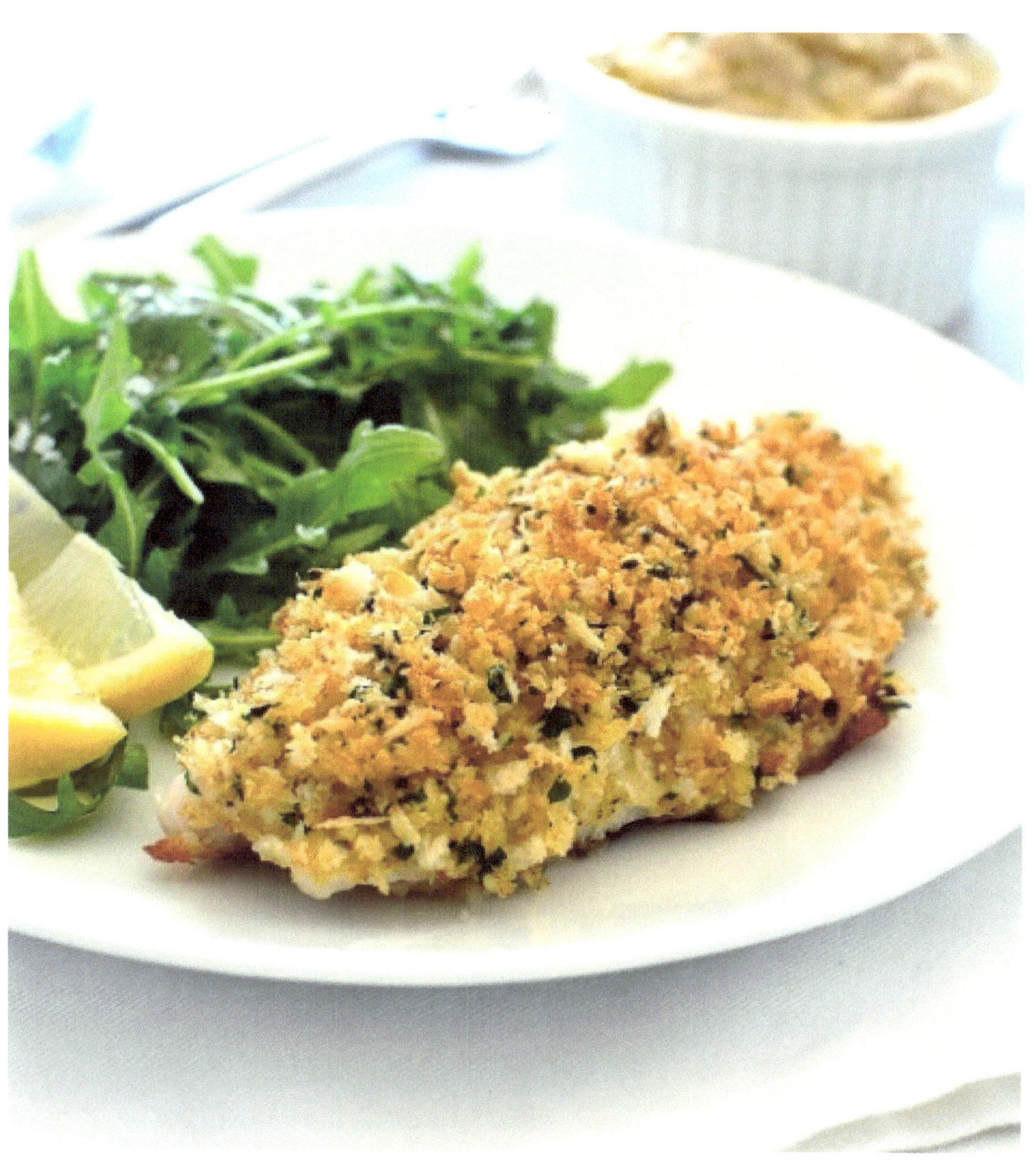

6)Almond Crusted Fish

Prep Time: 10 mins

Serves: 4

Ingredients:

- 1/2 cup raw almonds, chopped
- 1 garlic clove, chopped
- 4 white fish fillets
- 1 tsp. dried oregano
- 3 egg whites, beaten
- Pepper and salt to taste
- Green beans to serve

Directions:

- Preheat an oven to 375 F.

- Mix garlic, oregano, and almonds in a food processor or blender until a light crumb is formed.

- Mix in salt and black pepper and place on a plate.

- Whisk egg whites in another bowl. Dip each fish fillet in the beaten egg whites; gently roll it in the almond mixture.

- Place the coated fish on a lined baking tray; bake for 6-7 minutes each side.

- Serve with your favorite salad or green beans and lemon!

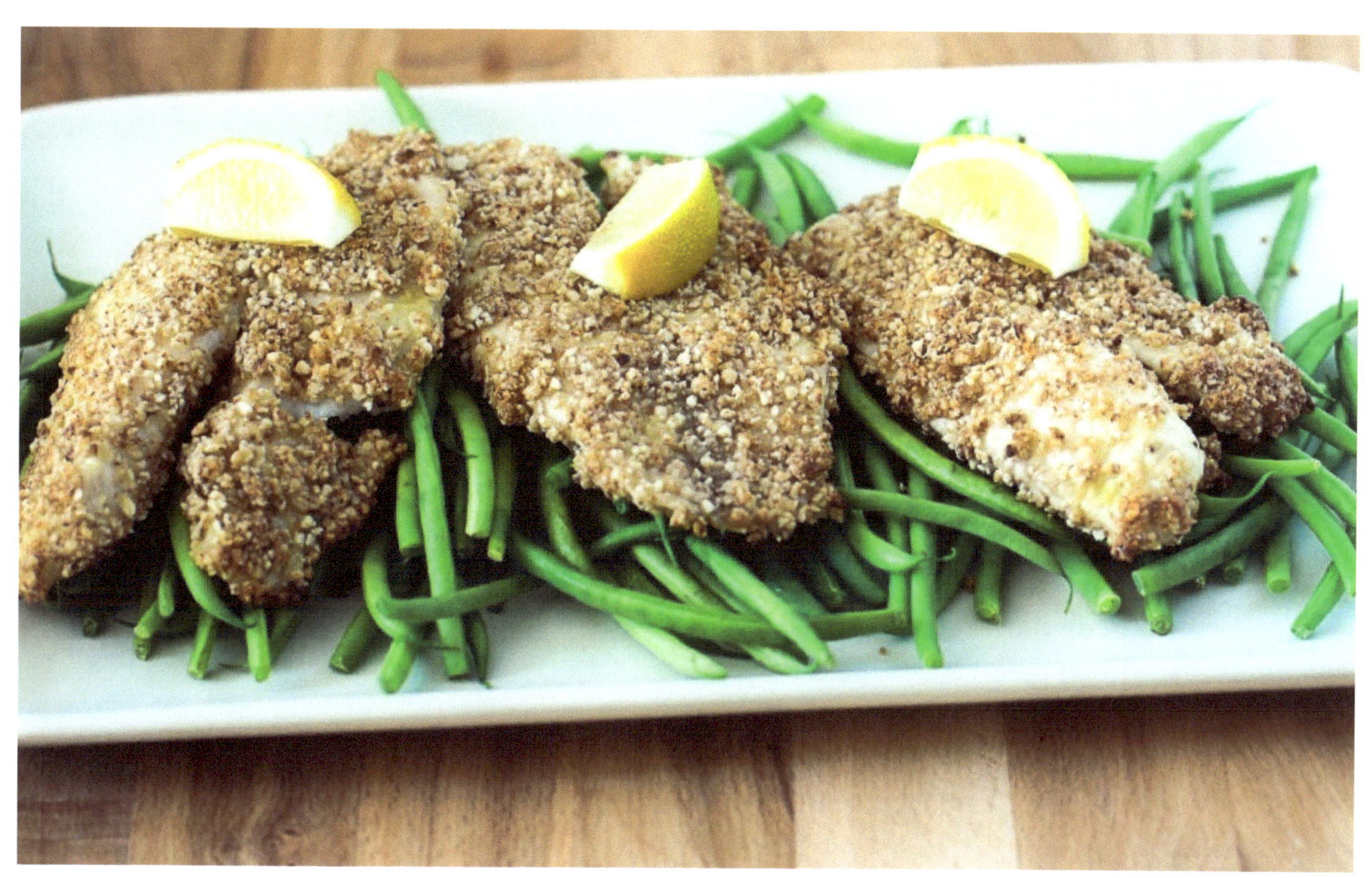

Chapter 2: Wholesome Mains

7) Refreshing Minty Lentil Spaghetti

Prep Time: 30-35 mins

Serves: 4-5

Ingredients:

- 1 can brown lentils, rinsed, drained
- 1 cup green olives, pitted and halved
- 2 garlic cloves, chopped
- 12 oz. spaghetti
- 1/2 onion, chopped
- 1 cup feta cheese, crumbled
- 3 tbs. extra virgin olive oil
- 1/3 cup fresh mint, finely cut
- 2 cups tomato sauce
- 2 cups water
- 1 tsp. salt

Directions:

- Heat a deep saucepan over medium-high heat.

- Add some oil and cook lentils, onion, garlic, olives, water, and tomato sauce.

- Boil the mixture.

- Add spaghetti and stir. Reduce heat and simmer until the spaghetti is cooked well.

- Top with some feta cheese and mint, adjust seasonings as required and serve.

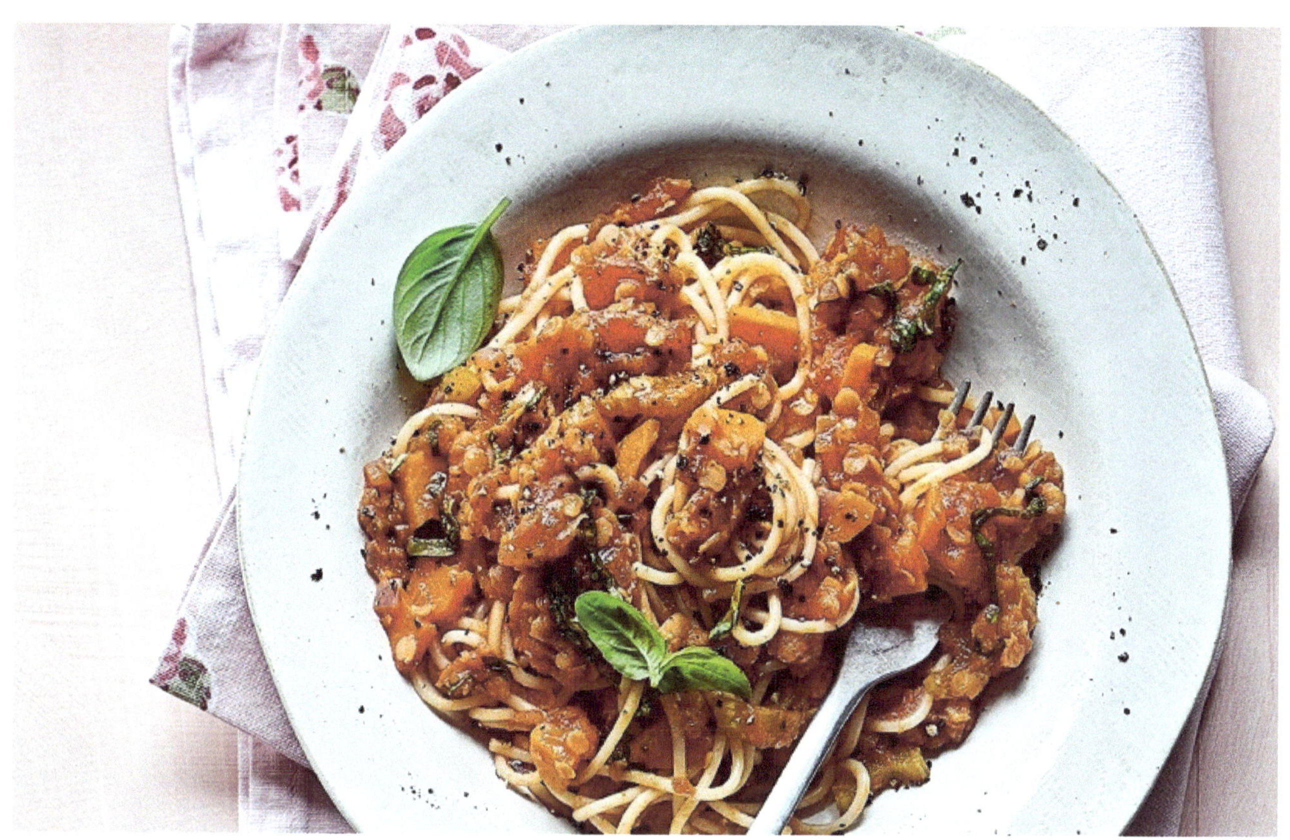

8) Chicken Avocado Spaghetti

Prep Time: 15-20 mins

Serves: 6

Ingredients:

- 2 avocados, peeled and diced
- 1 garlic clove, chopped
- 2 tbs. basil pesto
- 1 cup cherry tomatoes, halved
- 12 oz. spaghetti, whole wheat
- 1 cup cooked chicken, shredded
- 5 tbs. olive oil
- 4 tbs. lemon juice
- 1/4 cup grated Parmesan cheese

Directions:

- Take a large pot of boiling salted water; add the spaghetti.

- Cook, according to package instruction.

- Drain water and set aside in a large bowl.

- In a blender, mix lemon juice, garlic, basil pesto, and avocados; combine well until the ingredients are smooth.

- Mix the spaghetti, chicken, cherry tomatoes and avocado sauce on a serving plate.

- Top with some cheese and serve immediately.

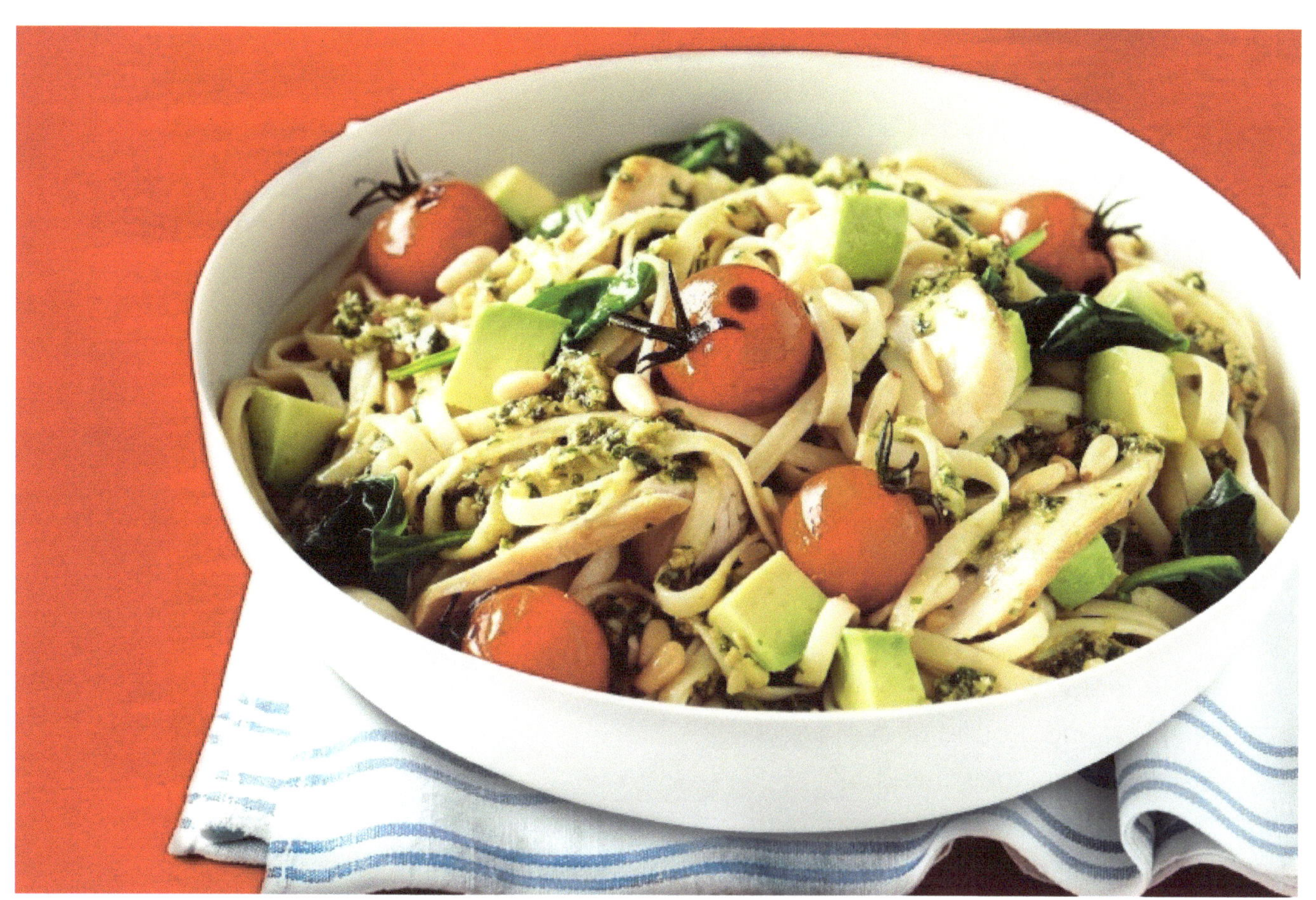

9) Quinoa Beef Casserole

Prep Time: 50-55 mins

Serves: 4-5

Ingredients:

- 1/2 pieced cabbage head, shredded
- 1 tomato, diced
- 1 tbs. paprika
- 1/2 tsp cumin
- 1/2 onion, chopped
- 2 leeks, white part only, chopped
- 1 pound ground beef
- 1 cup quinoa, rinsed
- 1/2 tsp. black pepper
- 4 tbs. extra virgin olive oil
- Salt as needed

Directions:

- In a medium size deep saucepan, sauté onion and leeks in olive oil until turn tender.

- Add in: beef, quinoa, tomato, paprika, cumin, pepper and salt. Stir very well.

- Add cabbage on the bottom of an ovenproof baking dish.

- Cover with beef and quinoa mixture.

- Cover it with aluminium foil and bake at 325 F for 38-40 minutes.

- Serve warm!

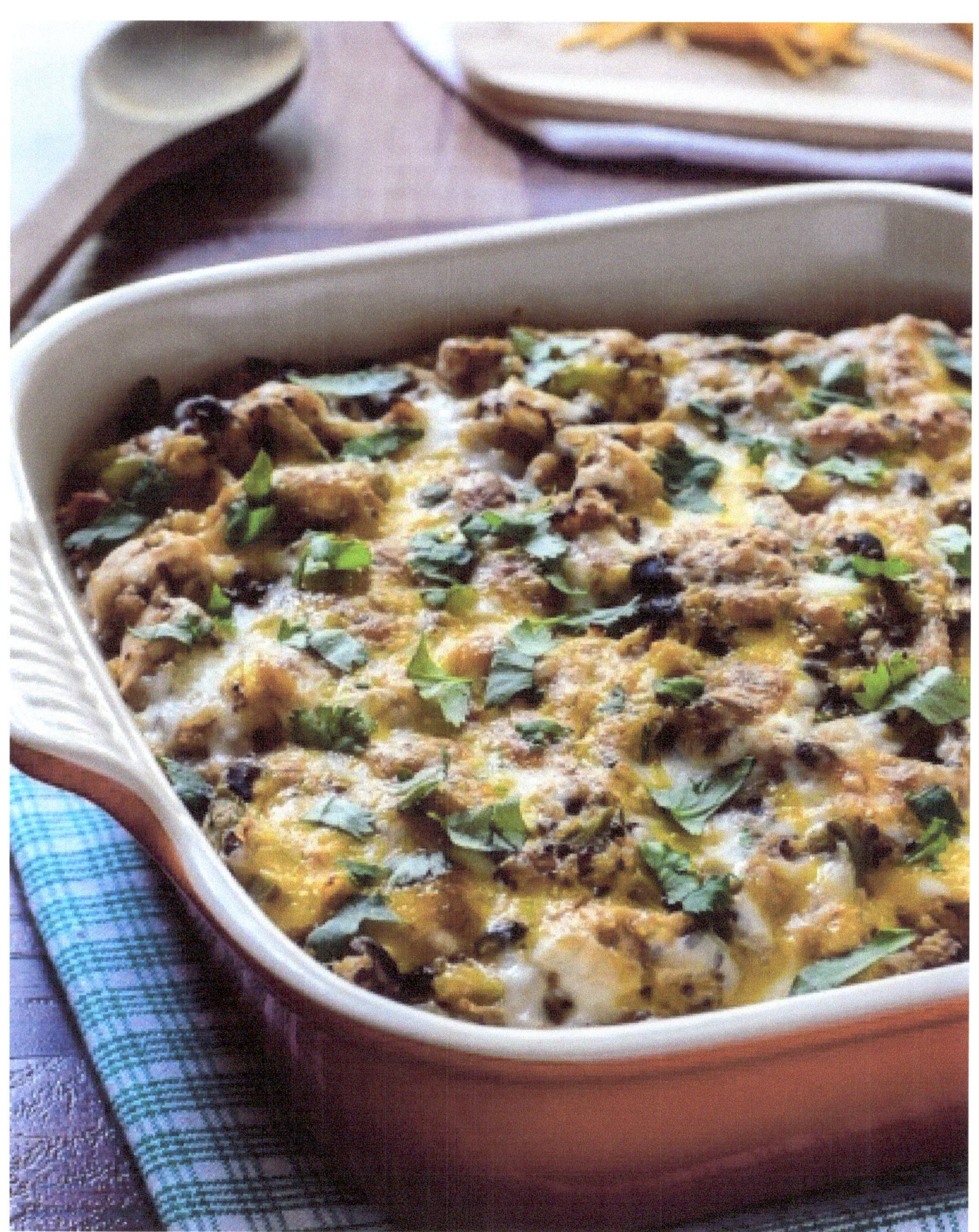

10) Arugula Corn Pasta

Prep Time: 8-10 mins

Serves: 4

Ingredients:

- 1 large avocado, peeled and diced
- 1 cup baby arugula leaves
- 3 cups cooked whole wheat pasta
- 3 tbs. olive oil
- 3 tbs. lemon juice
- 1/2 cup corn kernels, cooked
- 2 tbs. basil pesto
- 1/2 cup Parmesan cheese, grated

Directions:

- Thoroughly combine some olive oil, lemon juice, basil pesto and half the cheese in a small bowl.

- Season with salt and pepper.

- Mix the pasta, avocado, corn and baby arugula.

- Add the oil mixture and toss to combine.

- Serve with remaining cheese.

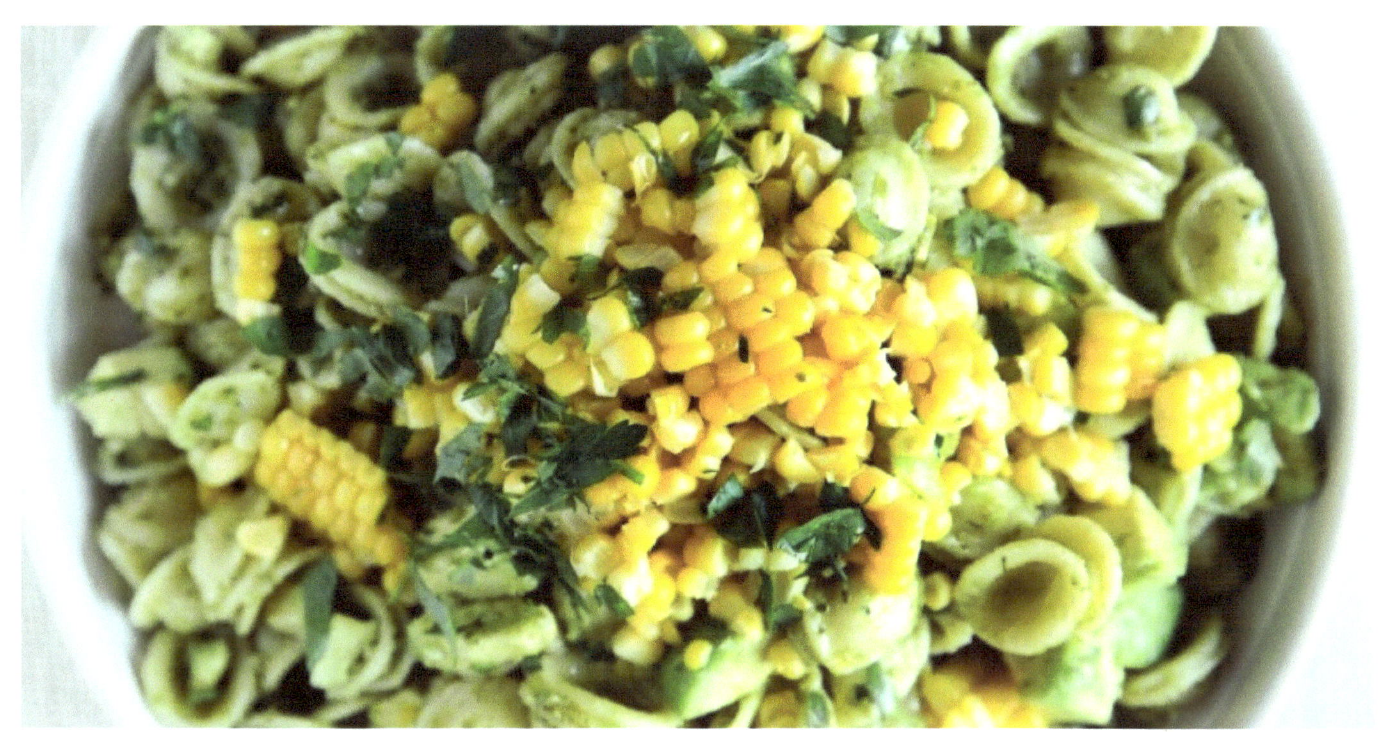

11)Wholesome Mushroom Chicken Meal

Prep Time: 30 mins

Serves: 4

Ingredients:

- 1 onion, chopped
- 4 tbs. extra virgin olive oil
- 4 chicken breasts, diced
- 2 pounds mushrooms, chopped
- 1 tbs. thyme
- 1 tbs. lemon rind
- Pepper and salt as needed

Directions:

- Heat some oil in a deep frying saucepan over medium-high heat.

- Add chicken, stirring, for 2 minutes each side, or until it turns evenly brown.

- Add onion, mushrooms, lemon rind, salt and black pepper and mix well.

- Reduce heat, cover, and simmer for 25-30 minutes.

- Remove cover and simmer for 5 minutes more.

- Serve warm!

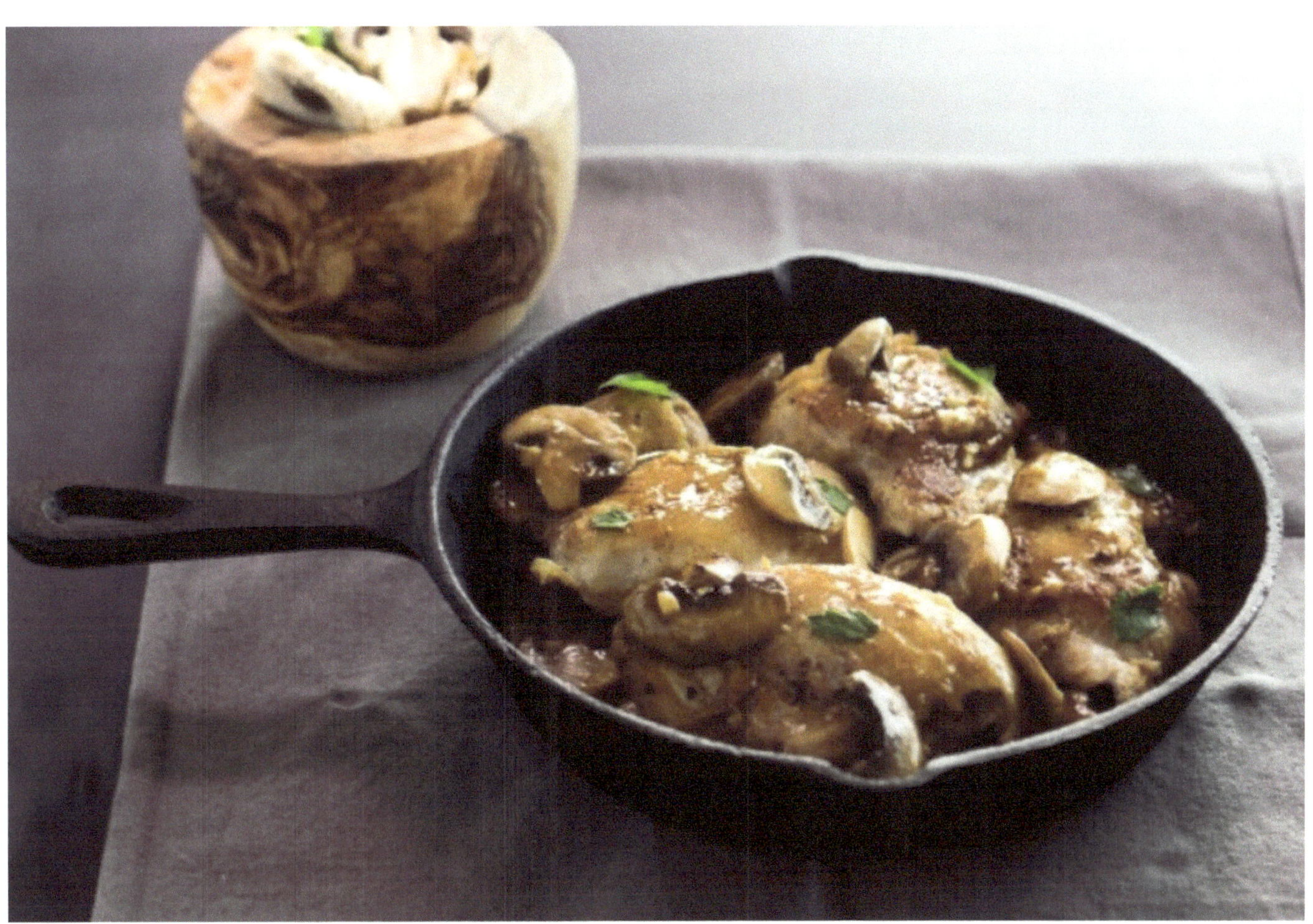

12) Bean Rice Casserole

Prep Time: 25-30 mins

Serves: 4

Ingredients:

- 2/3 cup rice
- 2 onions, chopped
- 2 cans (15 oz.) white or red beans, drained
- 1 cup vegetable broth
- 3 tbs. olive oil, extra virgin
- 1 tbs. paprika
- 1 cup parsley, finely cut
- 7-8 fresh mint leaves, finely cut
- 1/2 tsp. black pepper
- 1 tsp. salt

Directions:

- Heat some oil in a large saucepan.

- Add and gently sauté onions for 1-2 minutes.

- Mix paprika and rice and cook, stirring constantly, for 1minute.

- Add beans and vegetable broth, season with salt and pepper.

- Mix mint and parsley,

- Add the mixture on an ovenproof casserole dish.

- Bake in a preheated oven at 350 F for 20 minutes.

- Serve warm!

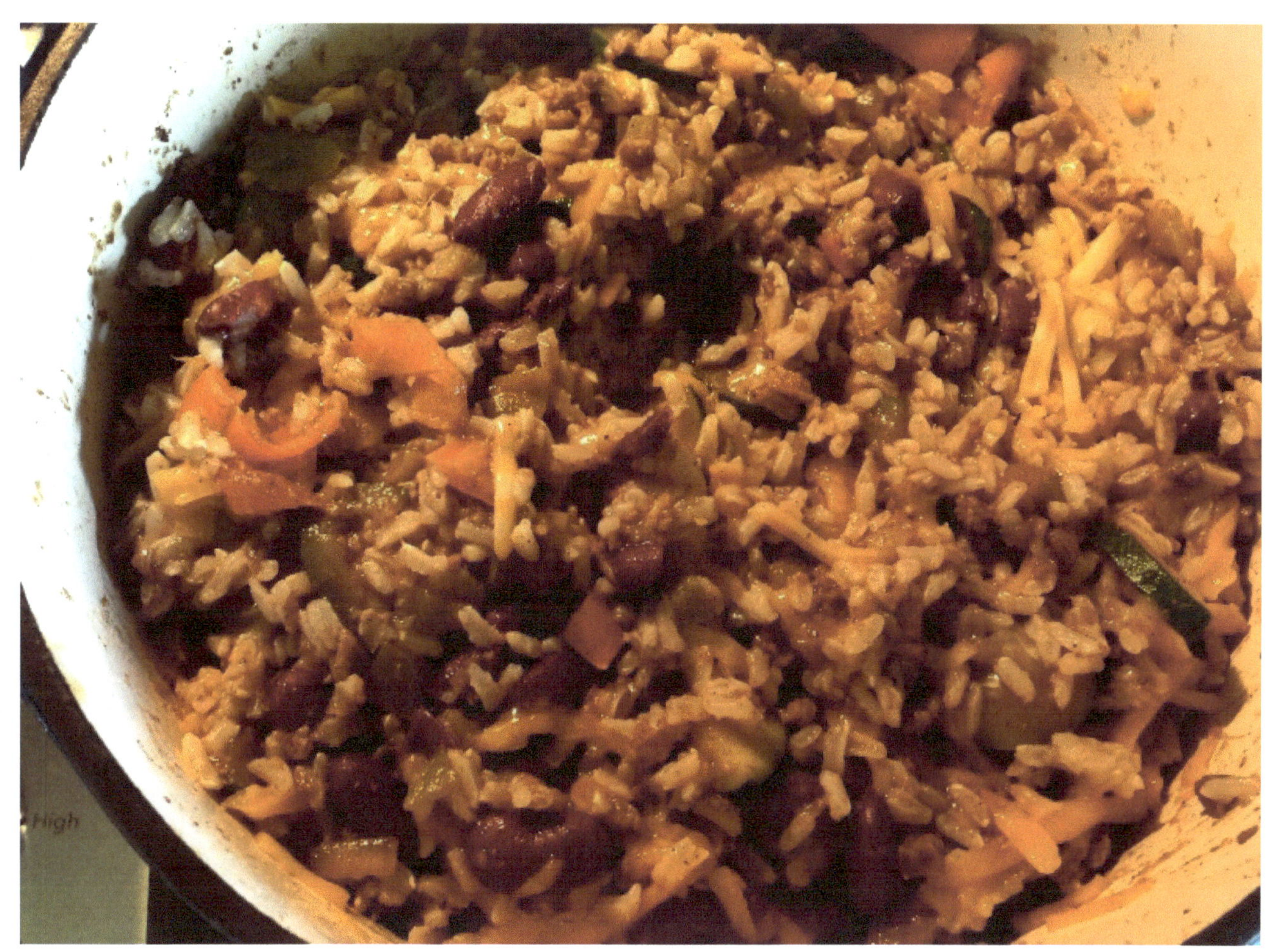
High

Chapter 3: Scrumptious Soups

13) Chickpea Bean Curry

Prep Time: 25-30 mins

Serves:4

Ingredients:

- 1 red onion, finely sliced
- 4 cups chickpeas, rinsed
- 1/2 cup low-fat plain yogurt
- 1 red capsicum, chopped
- 1/2 cup vegetable stock
- 1 cup green beans, halved
- 1 tbs. olive oil
- 2 garlic cloves, crushed
- 1 1/2 tsp. spice mix
- 1 long red chili, deseeded and chopped
- Whole meal pita bread for serving

Directions:

- In a medium saucepan, heat some oil over medium heat.

- Add chili, garlic, and onions; cook for 3-4 minutes to sauté.

- Add the spice mix, and capsicum cook for 2-3 minutes

- Add the stock, bean and chickpeas; boil the mixture

- Cover and simmer for 5 more minutes to soften the beans.

- Serve with warm pita bread and yogurt!

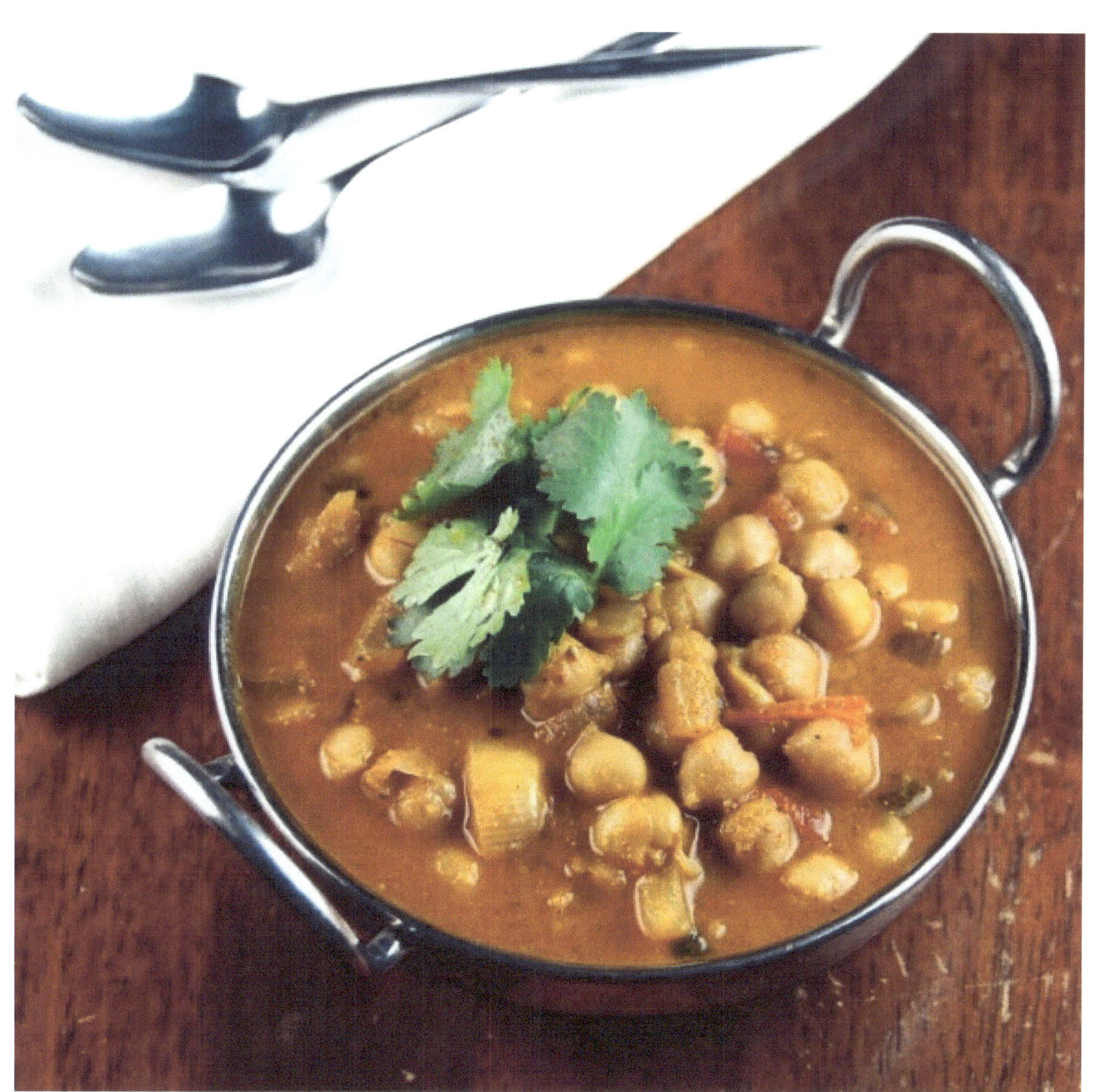

14) Prawn Avocado Soup

Prep Time: 15-20 mins

Serves: 8

Ingredients:

- 3 cups prawn stock
- 3 spring onions, chopped
- 3 pound cooked, peeled and deveined prawn
- 3 cups tomato juice
- 2 large tomatoes, diced
- 1 cup finely chopped parsley
- 3 avocados, peeled and diced
- 1 cucumber, peeled and diced
- 2 tbs. lime juice
- Pepper and salt to taste

Directions:

- Mix tomato juice and stock in a large bowl.

- Mix with prawns, avocados, cucumber, tomatoes, spring onions, parsley, lime juice, salt and pepper.

- Refrigerate until serving time.

- Serve chilled alone or with your favorite bread!

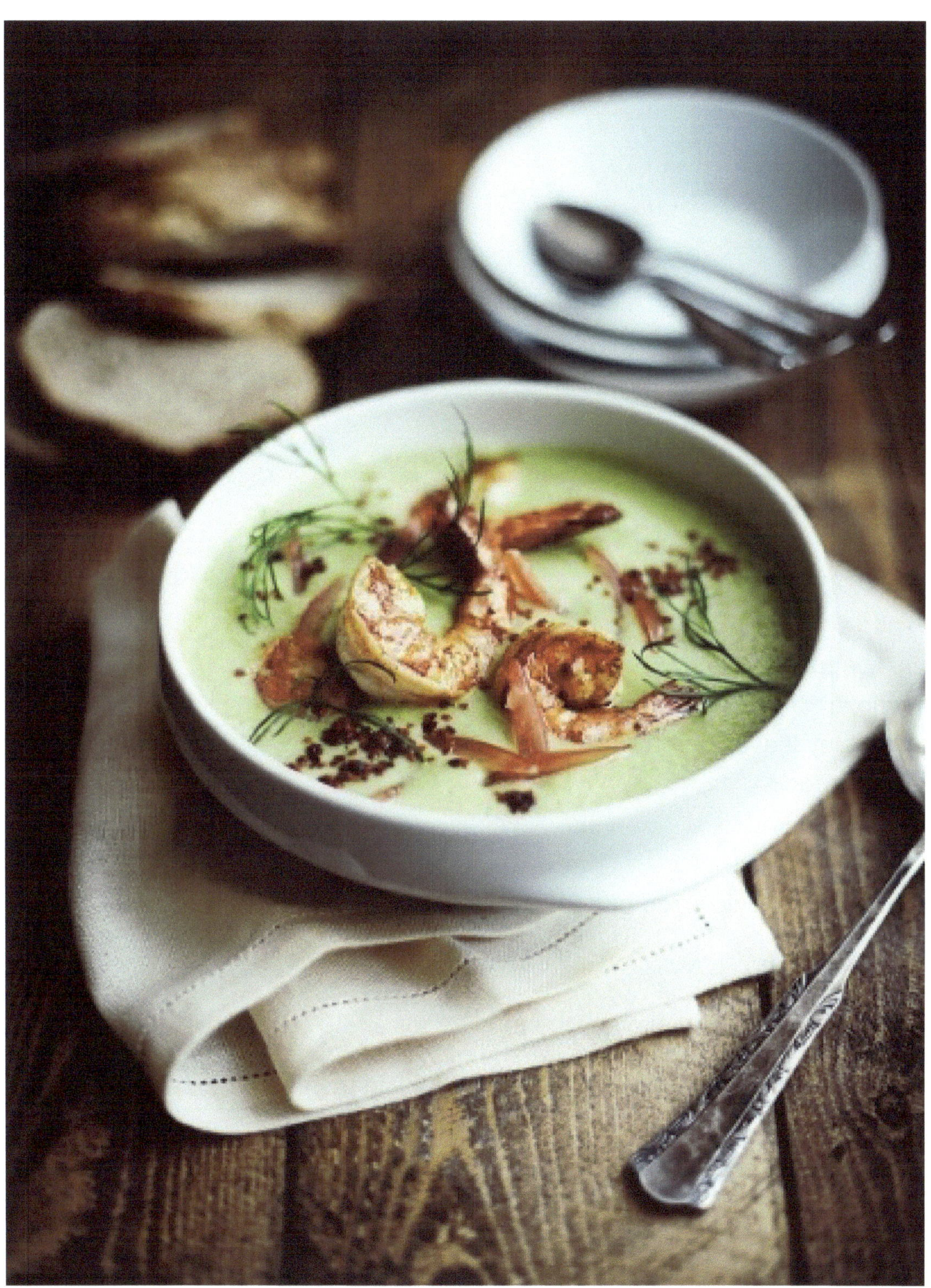

15) Chicken Oats Soup

Prep Time: 30-35 mins

Serves: 4

Ingredients:

- 3 garlic cloves
- 1/2 cup quick-cooking oats
- 1 large carrot, chopped
- 3 chicken breasts, diced
- 1 small onion, chopped
- 1 bay leaf
- 1 tsp. salt
- 1 red bell pepper, chopped
- 1 celery rib, chopped
- 1/2 cup parsley leaves, finely cut
- Pepper as needed

Directions:

- Add the chicken, carrot, onion, red pepper, bay leaf, celery, and salt into a pot.

- Add 6 cups of cold water.

- Bring to a boil, reduce heat and simmer the mixture for 25-30 minutes.

- Remove the bay leaf, season with salt and pepper; mix in the oats and parsley.

- Simmer for 4-5 more minutes, and serve.

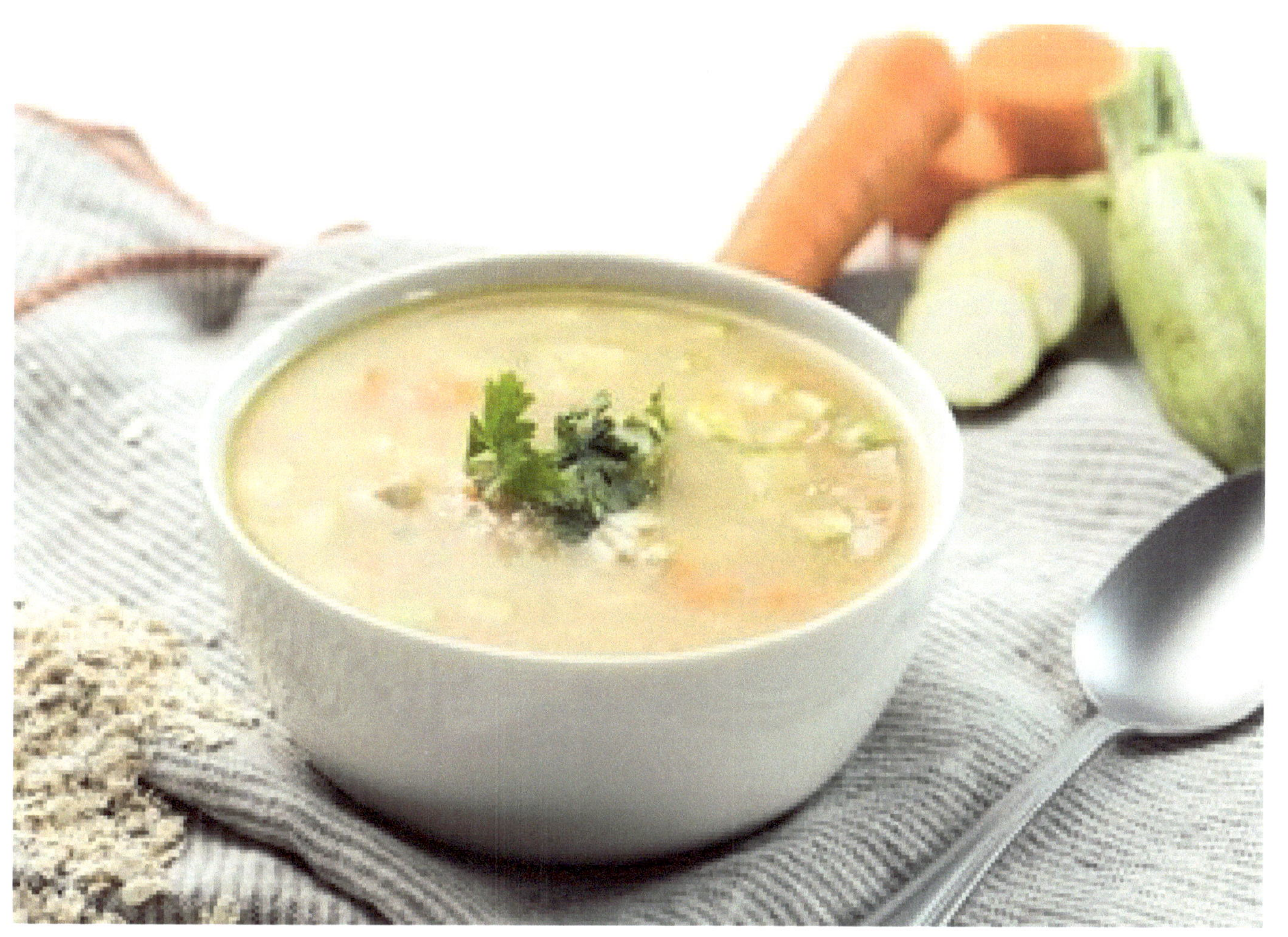

16) Spiced Quinoa Fish Soup

Prep Time: 25-30 mins

Serves:4-5

Ingredients:

- 3 tomatoes, chopped
- 1/2 cup quinoa, rinsed
- 1 red pepper, chopped
- 1 pound cod fillets, cubed
- ½ cup white wine
- 4 cups water
- 1/2 cup parsley, finely cut
- 1 onion, chopped
- 3 tbs. extra virgin olive oil
- A pinch of cayenne pepper
- 1 tsp. dried thyme
- 1 tsp. dried dill
- ½ tsp. pepper
- 1 bay leaf
- 1 carrot, chopped
- 1/2 cup black olives, pitted and sliced
- 1 garlic clove, crushed
- Pepper and salt to taste

Directions:

- Heat some olive oil over medium heat, add onion, red pepper, garlic, and carrot.

- Cook until turn tender.

- Mix in cayenne pepper, bay leaf, herbs, salt, and pepper.

- Add some wine, water, quinoa, and tomatoes; bring to a boil.

- Turn down the heat, and cover it.

- Cook for 10 minutes. Mix in olives and fish; cook for another 10 minutes.

- Stir in parsley and serve warm!

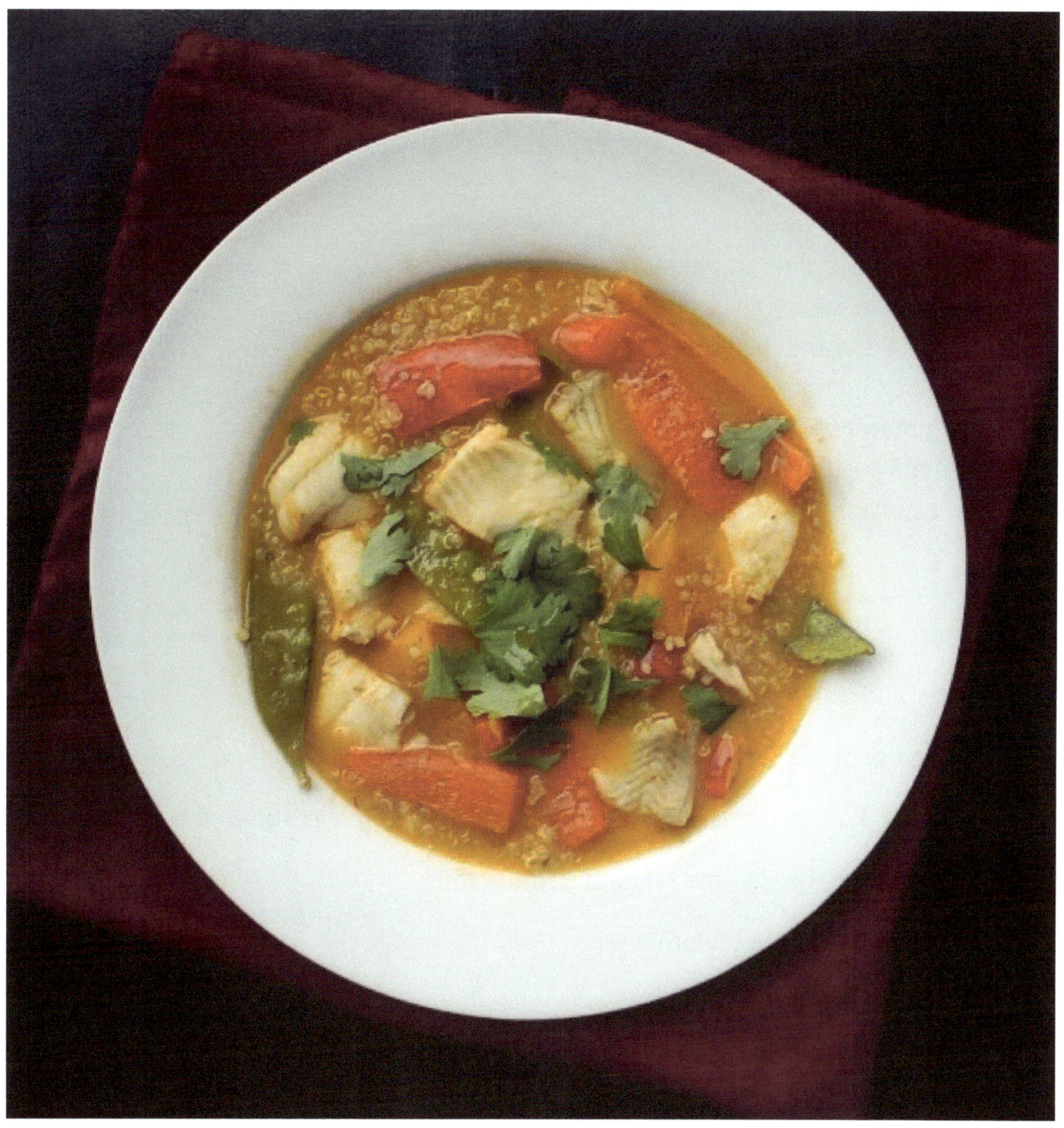

17) Tofu Bean Green Soup

Prep Time: 15-20 mins

Serves:4

Ingredients:

- 1 medium piece ginger, peeled and crushed
- 1/3 cup white miso paste.
- 4 stalks kale, remove stems
- 2 (7 or 8 oz.) packets udon noodles
- ½ cup green beans, trimmed
- 8 oz. marinated tofu, make small cubes
- 2 tsp. canola oil

Directions:

- In a saucepan, add 6 cups of water and heat it over high heat.

- Boil the water and add the miso; turn heat to medium.

- Add ginger and cook for 4-5 minutes.

- Add the noodles, kale and beans; cook for 6-7 more minutes to soften the noodles.

- In another saucepan, heat some oil, and add the tofu.

- Cook for 4-5 minutes to evenly brown

- Serve the soup with the tofu on top.

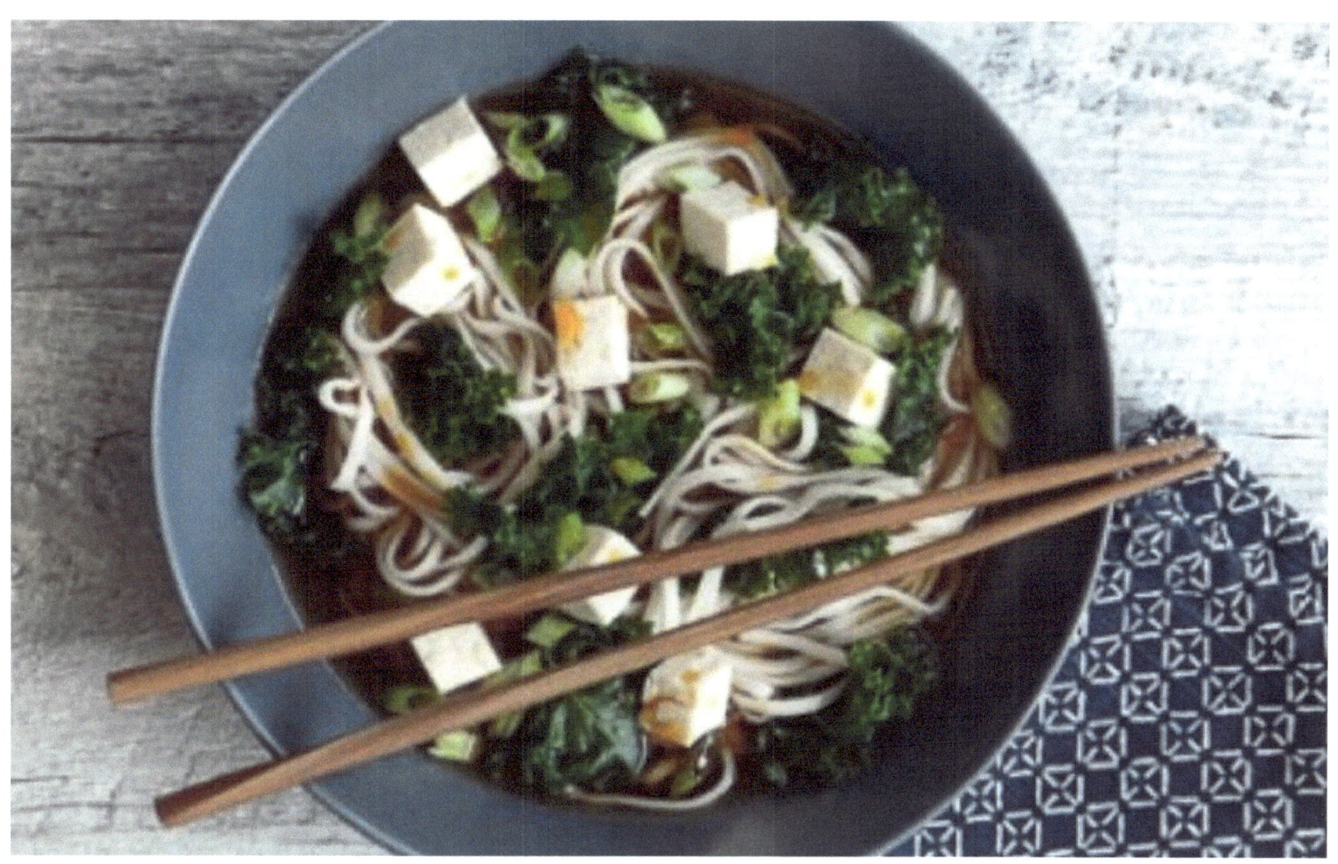

Chapter 4: Mouth Watering Healthy Desserts

18)Banana Chocolate Muffins

Prep Time: 15-20 mins

Serves: Makes 12 muffins

Ingredients:

- 1/2 cup milk
- 1/2 cup avocado, mashed
- 2 cups flour, all-purpose
- 1 cup sugar
- 2 eggs, large size
- 1/2 cup bananas, mashed
- 1 tsp. salt
- 1/2 cup chocolate chips
- 1 tsp. baking soda

Directions:

- Preheat an oven to 375 degrees F.

- Take 12 muffin tins and line with paper cups.

- In a large mixing bowl, combine eggs, bananas, avocado, and milk.

- In a separate bowl, thoroughly whisk soda, sugar, flour, and salt.

- Mix it with the avocado mixture and mix in the chocolate chips.

- Add the batter into muffin tins; bake 15-18 minutes or until top part becomes lightly brown.

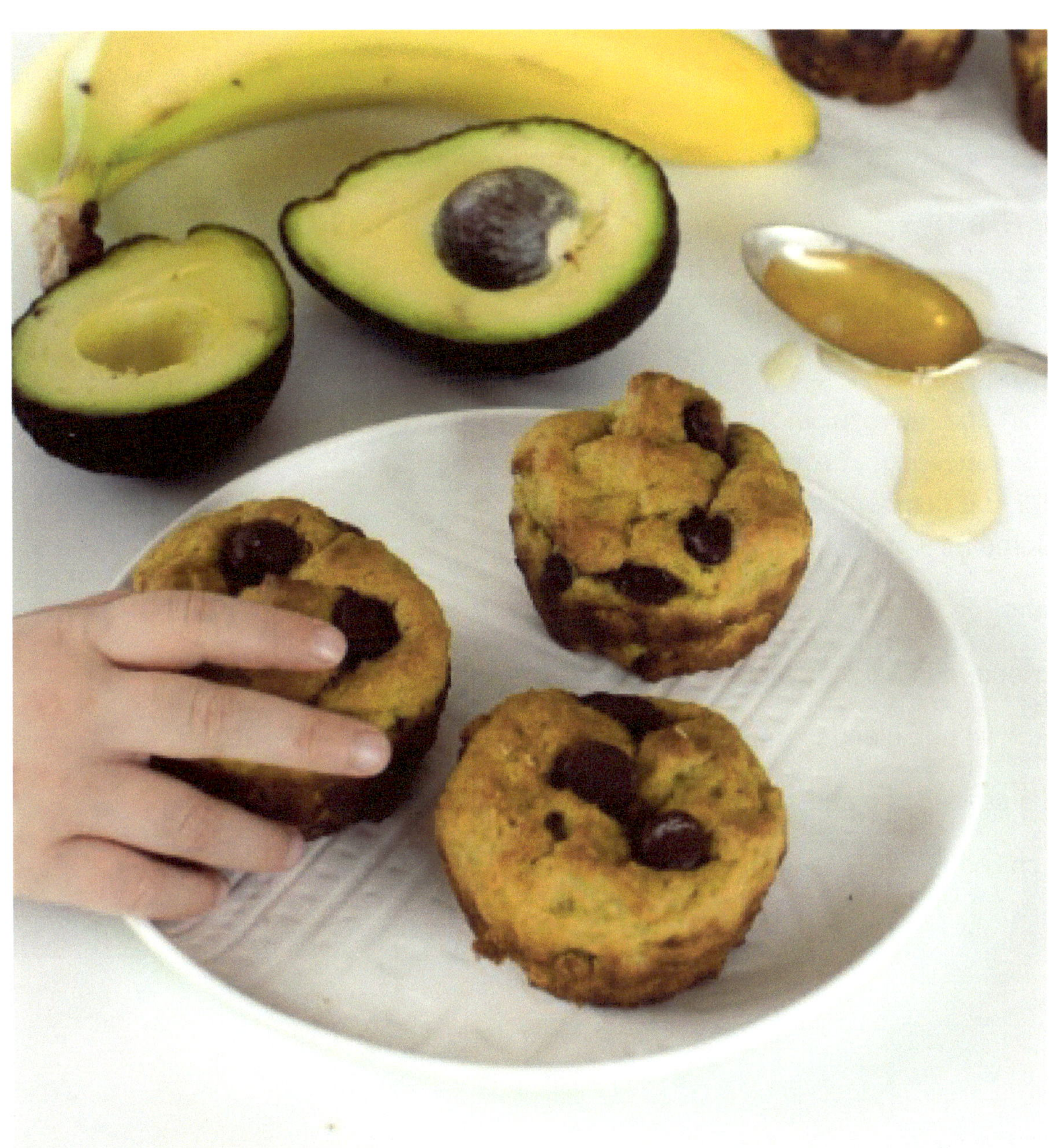

19)Mango Strawberry Sorbet

Prep Time: 8-10 mins

Serves: 2

Ingredients:

- 1/2 cup orange juice
- 1/2 cup mango, frozen
- 1/2 cup raspberries, frozen
- Some mint sprigs

Directions:

- One by one, add the ingredients in a blender.

- Close the lid and blend to make a smooth mixture.

- Add in a serving cup and add some mint leaves on top!

- Serve chilled!

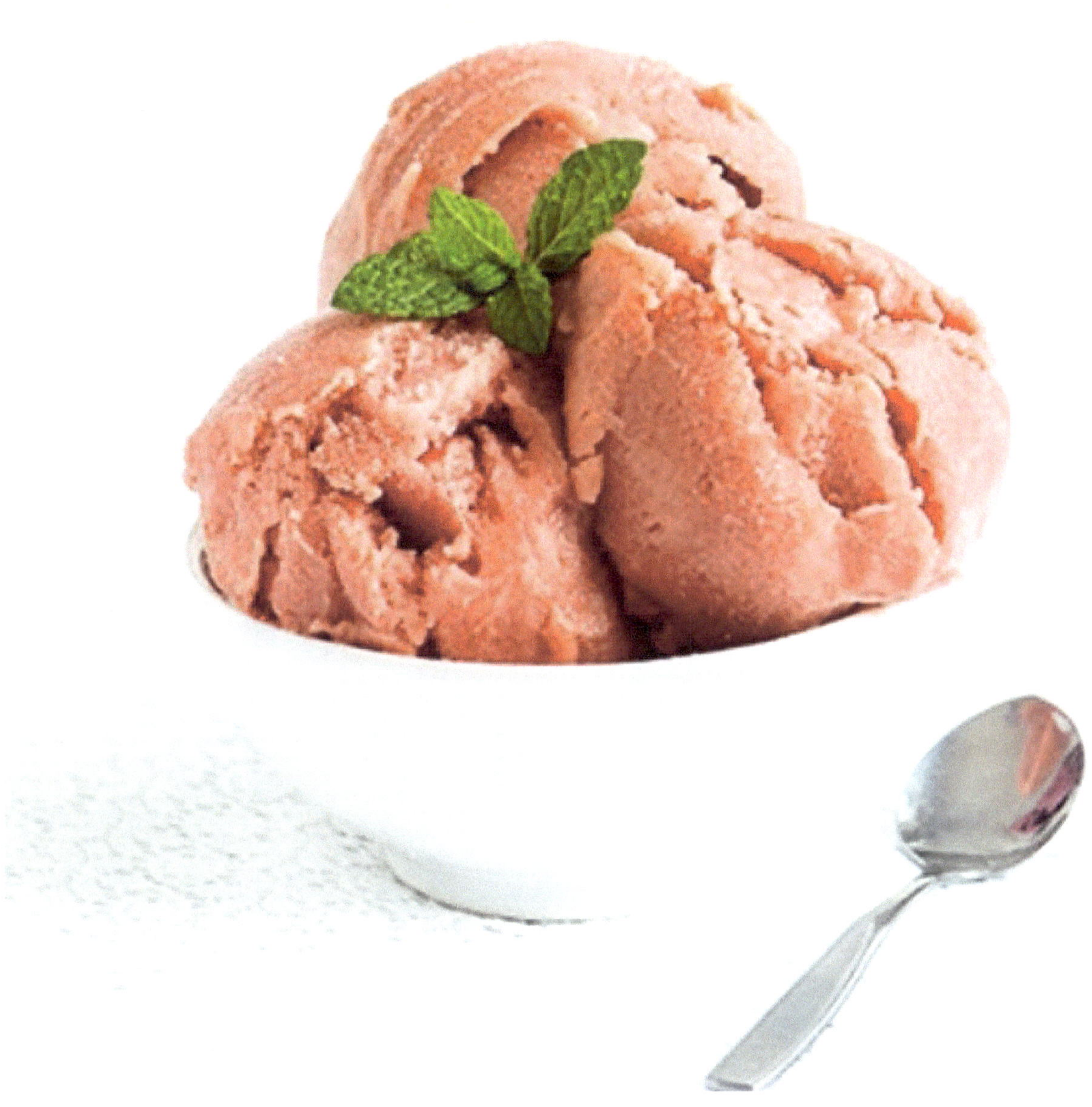

20)Cheesy Avocado Muffins

Prep Time: 20 mins

Serves: Makes 12 muffins

Ingredients:

- 1/4 cup sugar
- 3 eggs
- 1 cup flour, whole wheat
- 1 cup cornmeal
- 1 tsp salt
- 1 tsp. baking powder
- 1/3 cup avocado, mashed
- 1 cup milk
- 1/2 cup Cheddar cheese
- 1 tsp. baking soda

Directions:

- Preheat an oven to 375 degrees F.

- Take 12 muffin tins and line with paper cups.

- In a large mixing bowl whisk baking powder, sugar, cornmeal, flour, baking soda, and salt.

- In a separate bowl, thoroughly whisk milk, eggs, and avocado.

- Mix it with the avocado mixture.

- Now mix in cheese.

- Add the batter into prepared muffin tins.

- Bake 15-18 minutes or until top part becomes lightly brown.

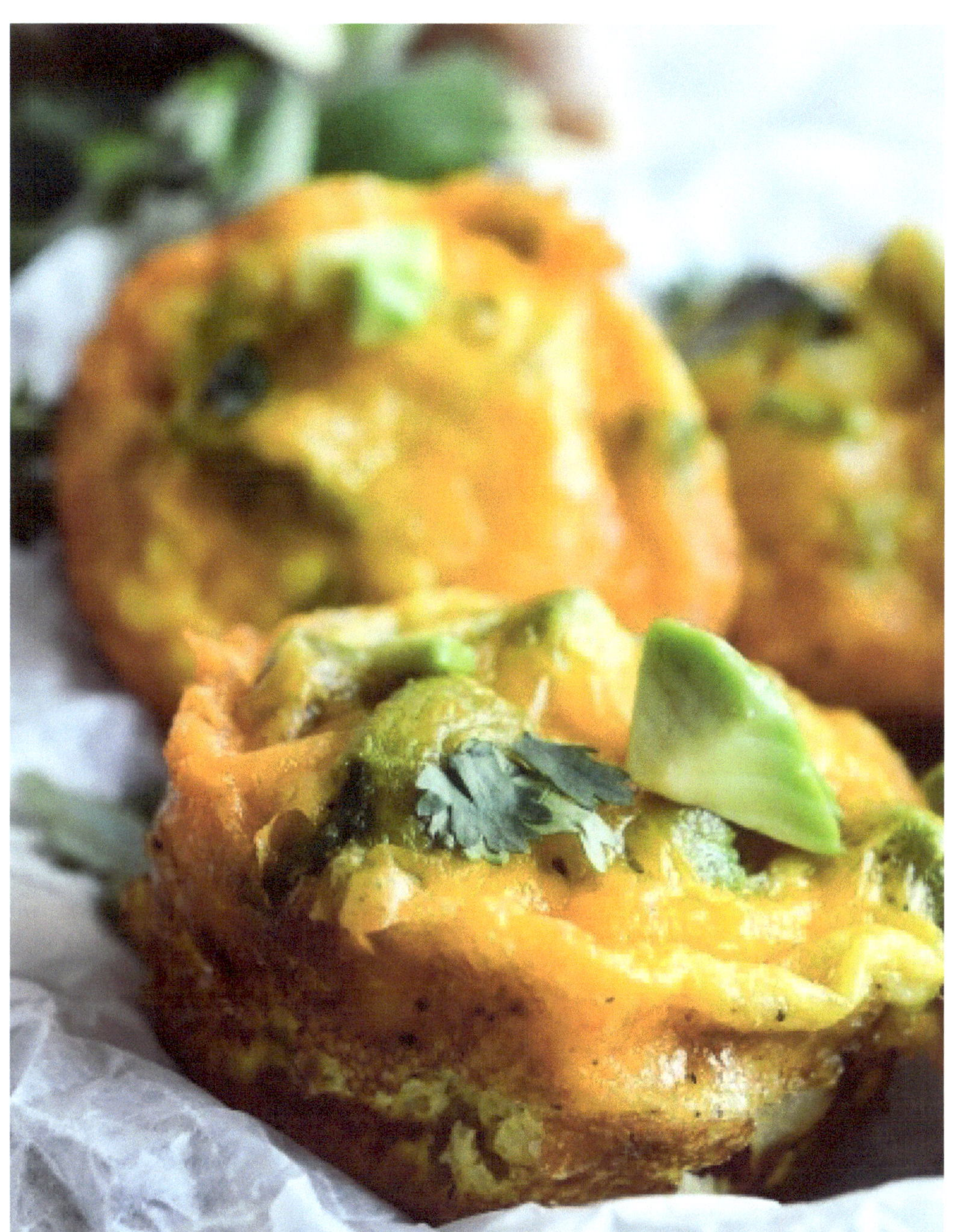

21) Cranberry Banana Pudding

Prep Time: 15 mins

Serves: 2

Ingredients:

- 3 tbs. flaked unsweetened coconut
- 4 tbs. maple syrup or honey
- 4 tbs. chia seeds
- 2 ripe bananas, chopped
- 2 cups coconut milk, low fat
- 1 tsp. vanilla extract
- 3 tbs. dried cranberries
- 2 tbs. walnuts, crushed

Directions:

- In a mixing bowl, whisk milk, honey or syrup, and vanilla.

- Add in chia seeds and flakes and let sit for 10 minutes.

- Whisk again, cover the bowl, and chill in the fridge for 3 hours, or overnight.

- Add into serving bowls and stir in banana.

- Top with some walnuts and cranberries.

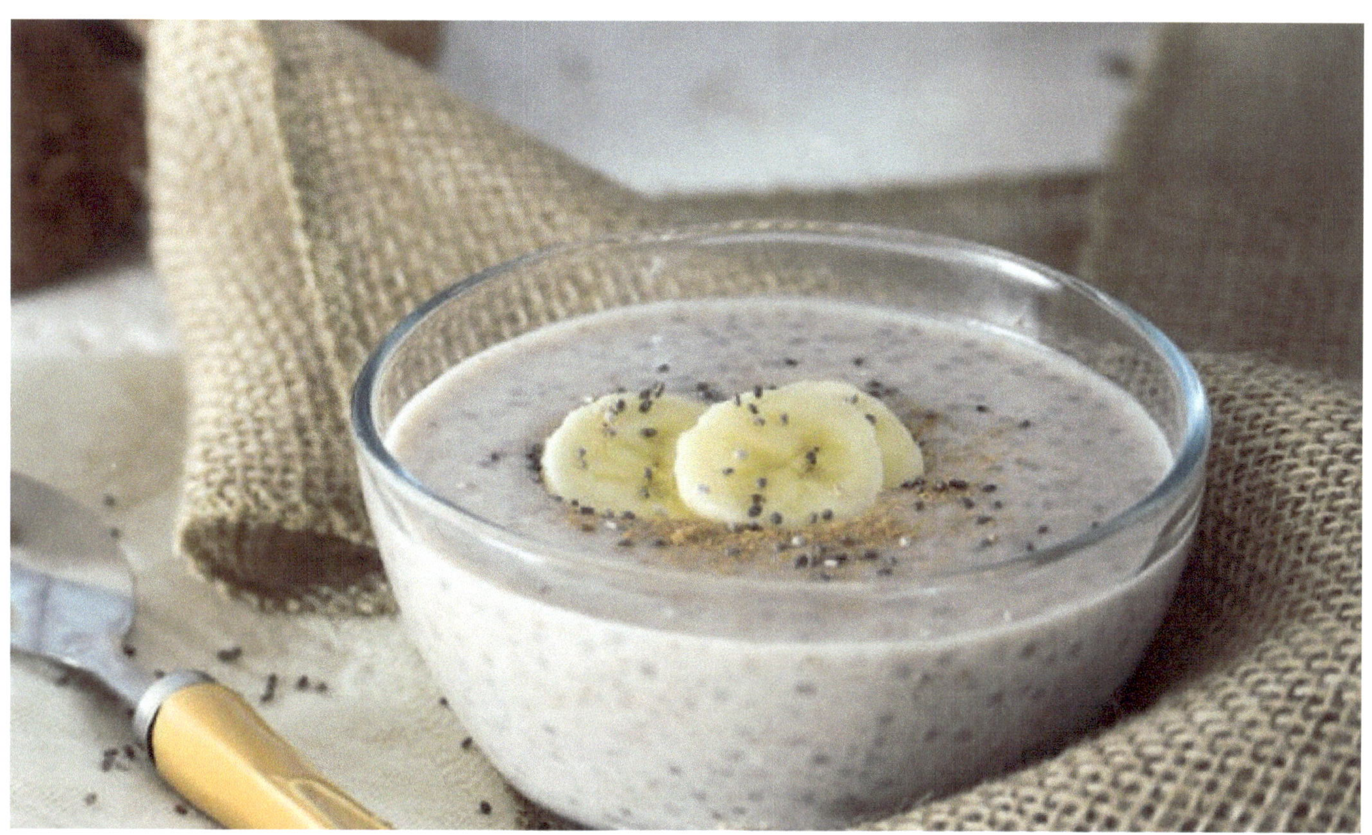

Chapter 5: Heart Healthy Drinks

22) Spinach Apple Juice Drink

Prep Time: 5 mins

Serves: 2-3

Ingredients:

- 1 cup raw spinach leaves
- 4 medium red apples
- 1 handful of parsley
- 3-4 ice cubes (optional)

Directions:

- Take your juicer and place it on a kitchen platform.

- One by one, juice all the ingredients and collect the juice in a container.

- Pour into serving glasses and add some ice cubed, if desired.

- Enjoy this healthy drink!

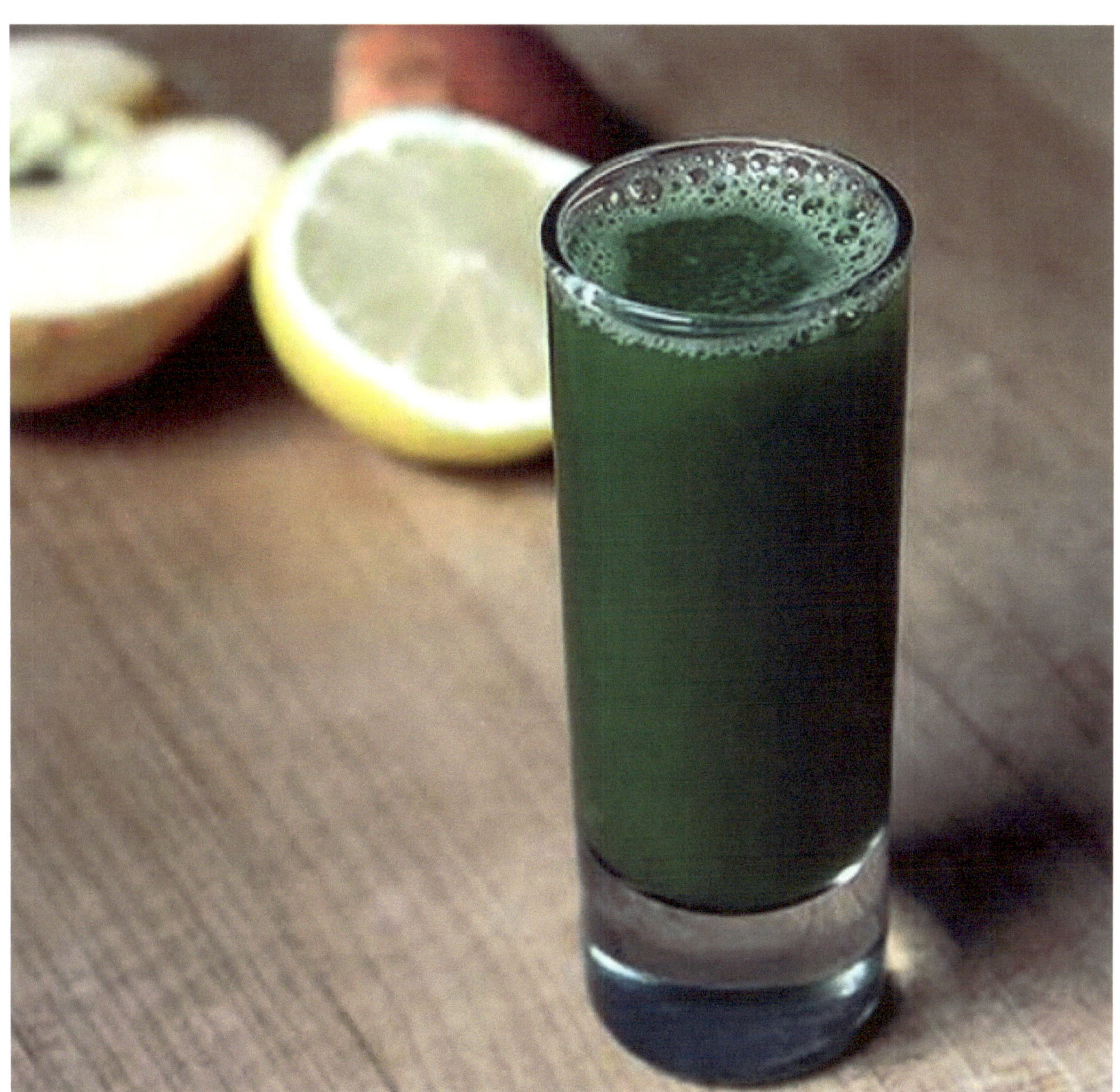

23) Kiwi Strawberry Drink

Prep Time: 5 mins

Serves: 2

Ingredients:

- 1 peeled kiwi
- 2 oranges
- 1 cup strawberries
- 3-4 ice cubes (optional)

Directions:

- Take your juicer and place it on a kitchen platform.

- One by one, juice all the ingredients and collect the juice in a container.

- Pour into serving glasses and add some ice cubed, if desired.

- Enjoy this healthy drink!

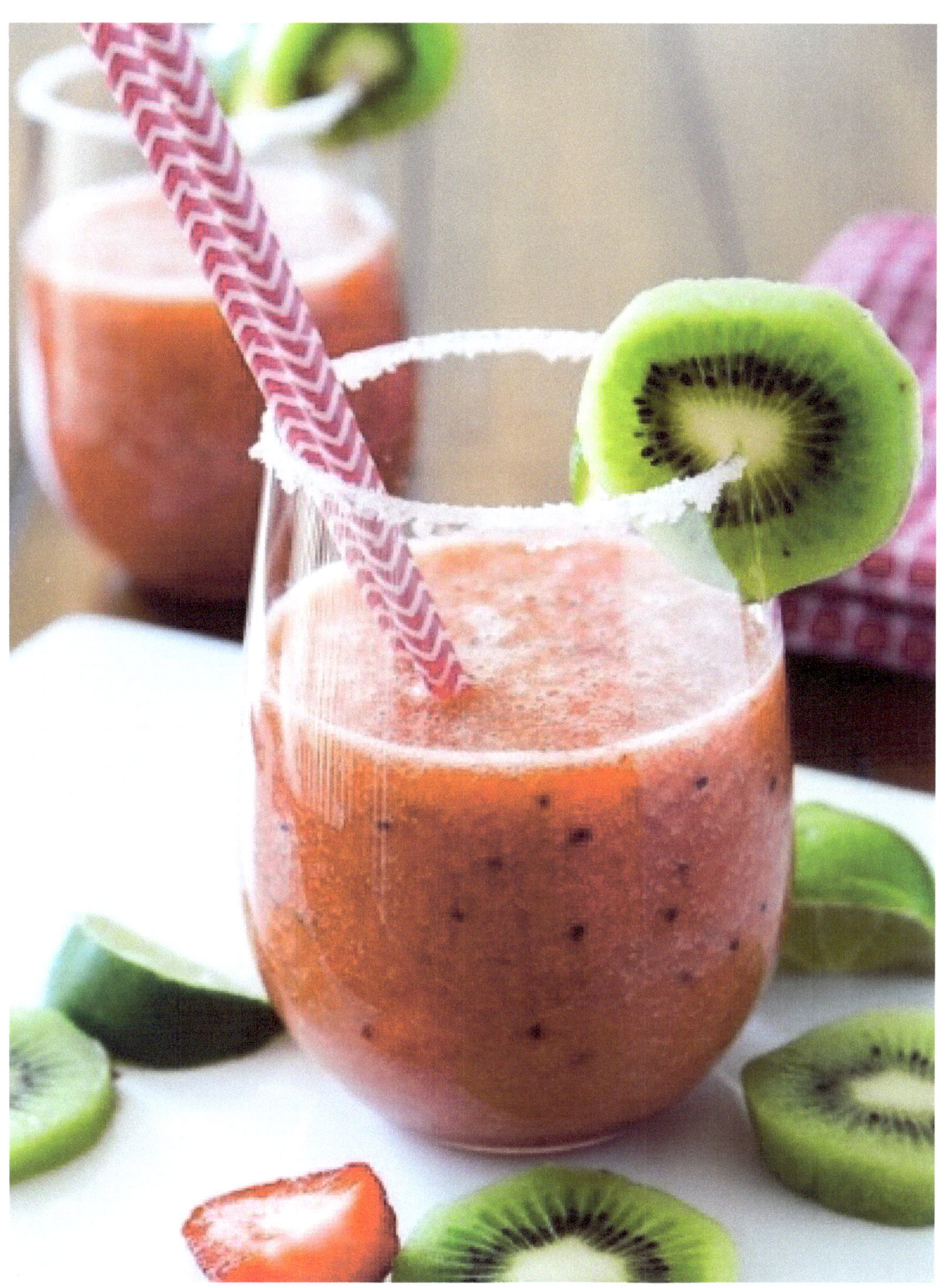

24) Coconut Strawberry Smoothie

Prep Time: 5 mins

Serves: 2-3

Ingredients:

- 3 cups strawberries
- 2 cups coconut milk
- 1 medium avocado, peeled and make cubes
- 4 ice cubes

Directions:

- One by one, add all the ingredients in a blender.

- Close the lid and blend until you get a smooth mixture.

- Add in a tall serving glass and enjoy this wholesome smoothie!

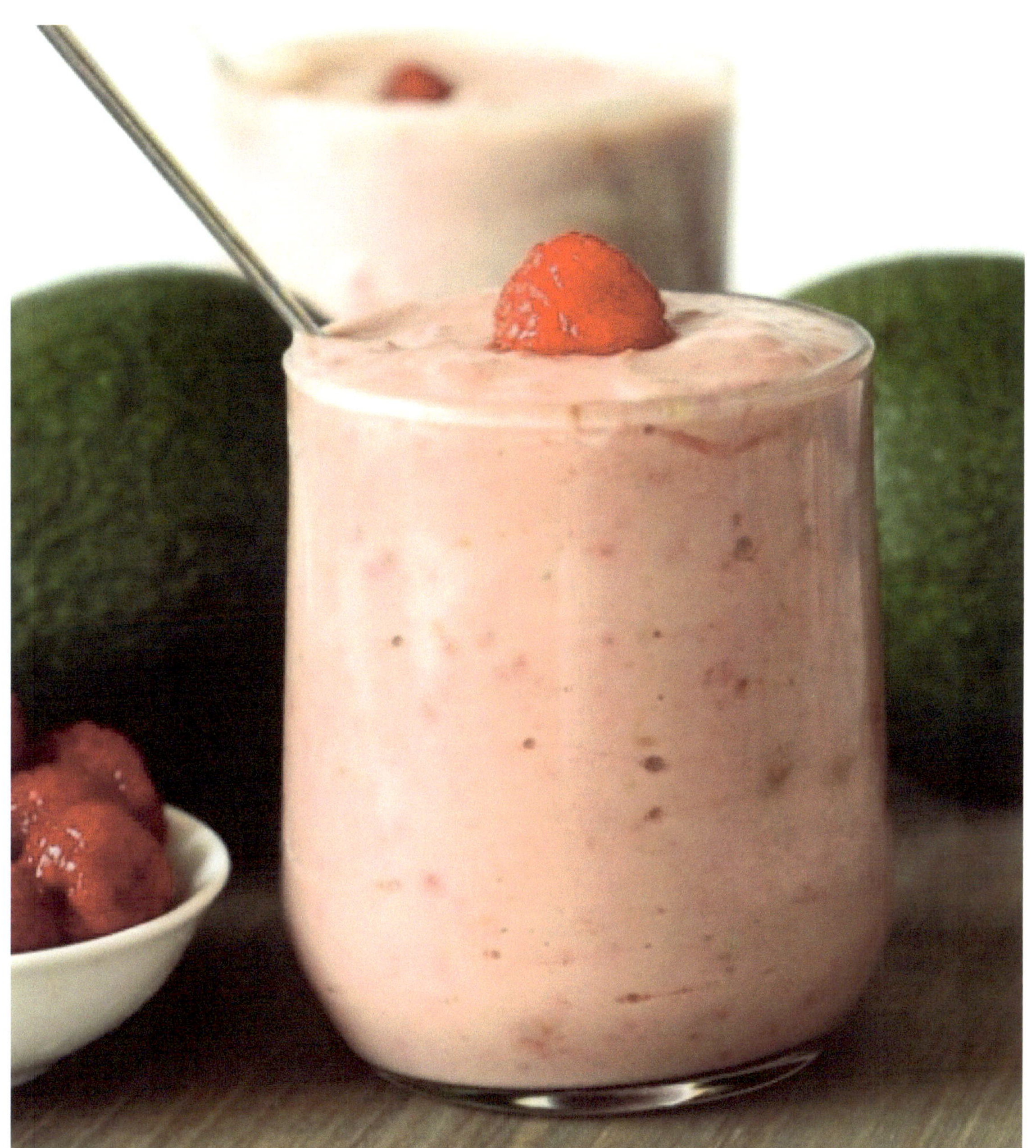

25) Green Apple Avocado Smoothie

Prep Time: 5-8 mins

Serves: 2-3

Ingredients:

- 3-4 ice cubes
- 3 green apples, peeled and chopped
- 1 cup parsley leaves
- 1 peeled avocado, chopped
- 1 cup orange juice
- Juice of 1 medium lime

Directions:

- One by one, add all the ingredients in a blender.

- Close the lid and blend until you get a smooth mixture.

- Add in a tall serving glass and enjoy this wholesome smoothie!

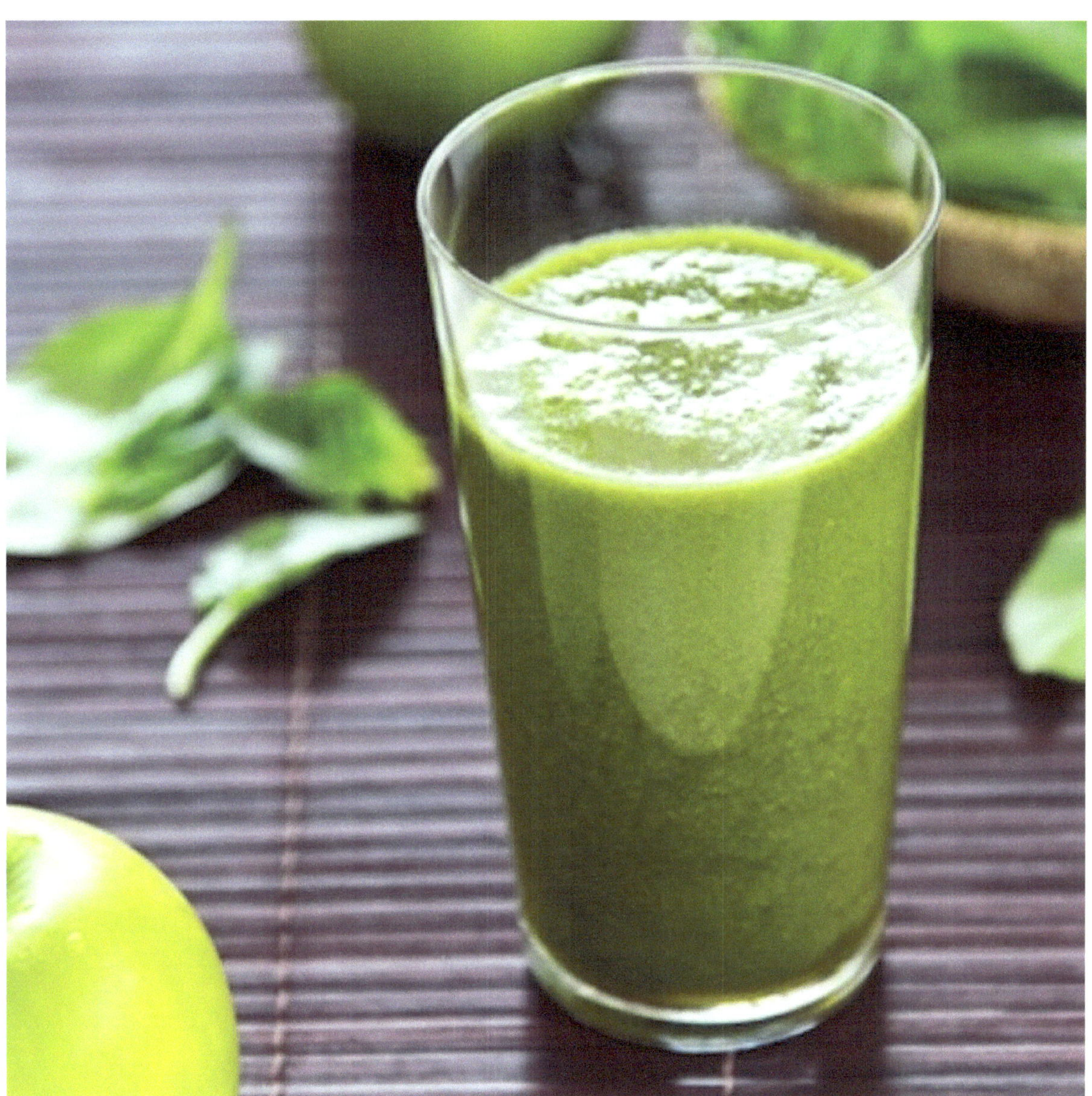

26) Avocado Mango Smoothie

Prep Time: 5-8 mins

Serves: 2-3

Ingredients:

- 1 cup carrot juice
- 1/2 cup orange juice
- 1 1/2 cups frozen mango chunks
- 1 avocado, peeled and chopped
- 1 tsp. grated ginger

Directions:

- One by one, add all the ingredients in a blender.

- Close the lid and blend until you get a smooth mixture.

- Add in a tall serving glass and enjoy this wholesome smoothie!

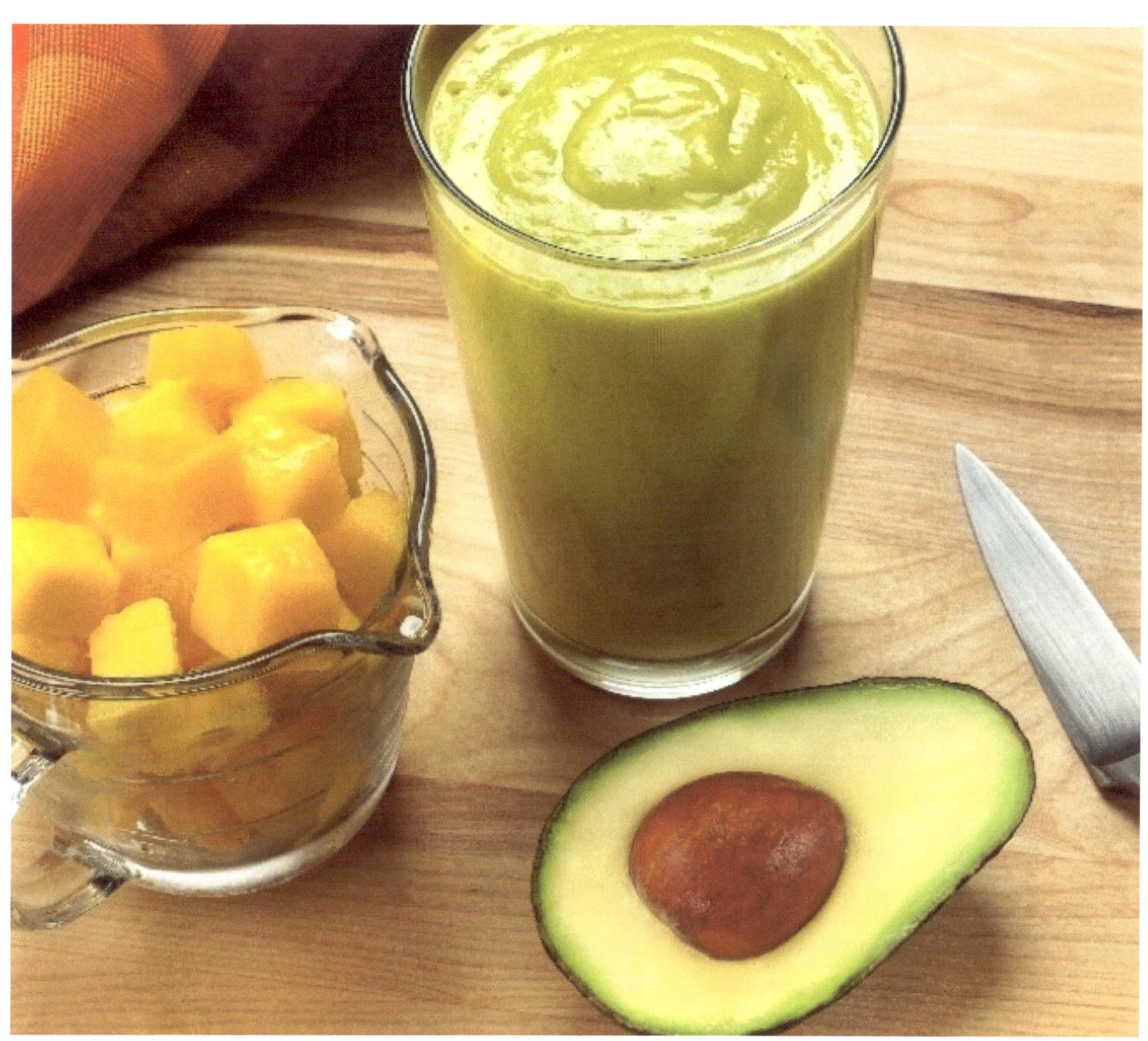

Conclusion

A healthy diet is a simple and straightforward solution to keep cholesterol levels in check. Apart from diet, regular exercise and relaxed sleep at night also play a vital role in keeping your heart healthy. You just need to replace some ingredients that can keep your cholesterol in check and avoid consuming certain ingredients that can spike up your cholesterol level.

Easy and delicious family-friendly recipes covered in the book aims at educating our readers to prepare healthy meals at home and control their cholesterol level. Dedicated efforts have been made to provide its readers with the most versatile collection of recipes to easily made at home and enjoy their health benefits.

We would like to thank all our readers to give their valuable time in reading this book. We sincerely hope that the recipes covered in this book will guide you in leading a truly healthy lifestyle and keep your heart young forever.

Experiment with the recipes by adding your favorite heart-friendly ingredients and create your own customized low cholesterol recipes.

Finally, if you enjoyed this dedicated book, please take a few minutes of your valuable time to share your views and suggestion at -- email address --. It'd be greatly appreciated!

Thank you again; good luck!

Happy healthy eating!

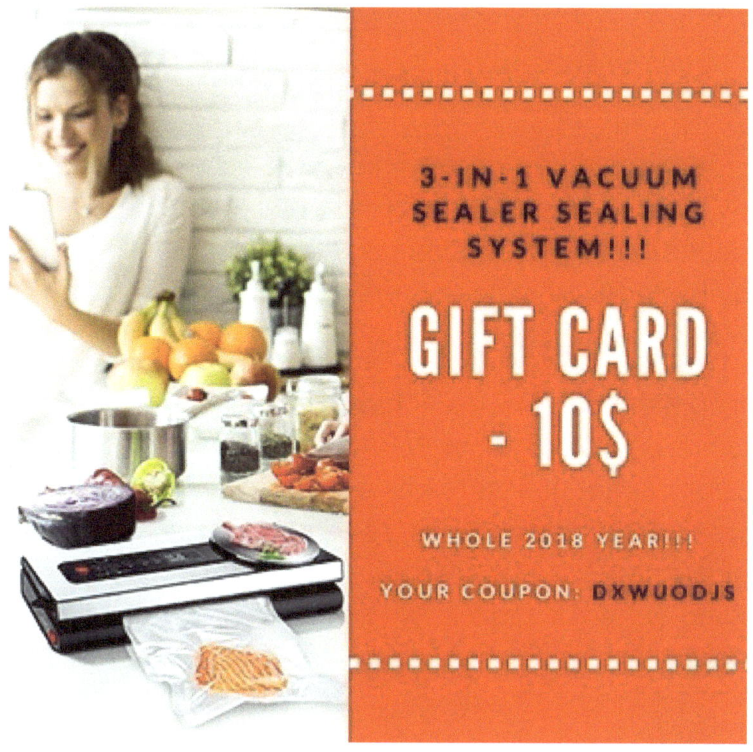

To our customers we give a discount to $10,

it's very easy to get it, use the coupon code

on the link

HERE

I know you will love this gift.

If you like this book, you can see and buy my other books on this link:

All books Jessica Huston here